FIGHTING
FOR *Taylor*

FIGHTING
FOR *Taylor*

*A Mother and Child's Journey
of Inclusion*

Kimberly Moore

iUniverse, Inc.
Bloomington

FIGHTING FOR TAYLOR
A Mother and Child's Journey of Inclusion

The following story is based solely on my memories. To protect the privacy of others, names of people and places have been changed and characters conflated.

iUniverse books may be ordered through booksellers or by contacting:

iUniverse
1663 Liberty Drive
Bloomington, IN 47403
www.iuniverse.com
1-800-Authors (1-800-288-4677)

Because of the dynamic nature of the Internet, any web addresses or links contained in this book may have changed since publication and may no longer be valid. The views expressed in this work are solely those of the author and do not necessarily reflect the views of the publisher, and the publisher hereby disclaims any responsibility for them.

Edited by: Alexander Malanych
Alison Pierce Photography for the back cover
alison@alisonpiercephotography.com

ISBN: 978-1-4759-5772-3 (sc)
ISBN: 978-1-4759-5774-7 (hc)
ISBN: 978-1-4759-5773-0 (ebk)

Library of Congress Control Number: 2012920567

Printed in the United States of America

iUniverse rev. date: 11/20/2012

Contents

Introduction 2012

It's a beautiful, humid rainy August summer day as I sit on my front porch watching the drops of water drip delicately from our American flag, proudly waving on a small pole in front of our little townhouse. Taylor is at a local agricultural fair with his favorite babysitter, allowing me to spend the day working. Every hour or so a ping from my Blackberry sounds as the sitter sends me a text message with a photo attached so I can see what he's up to, and all of the fun he's having—consoling my guilt as a mother for not being there with him while I work away my day.

The road to Vermont has been an arduous one, no doubt. From wealth to welfare, from despair to triumph, and from selfishness to compassion, I have lived life's every day challenges with hope and resilience, holding onto my dream for a better tomorrow. As I sit and relish the solitude of our front porch, my gratitude is greater than ever for the life my son has taught me to embrace. And for the first time, I have found peace as a parent and actually know its true meaning from deep within. What a remarkable country the United States of America is, and how blessed I am to live in a country where you can change the course of your life just by having a thought, a dream, and the ability to work hard.

It's been eight years of putting my pen to paper and telling the most intimate, personal parts of my son and I's life in the hopes of making a difference, even if to help only one person. This book is not just a personal account of a mother and child's journey; it is a call to action for all individuals who share a concern for education and social welfare, as well as parents who worry for their children's future, and their own. And it all begins at home. From my home to yours, I hope to instill thoughts and ideas about making tomorrow better for everyone; most of all, our kids. My son may be a little different and I may not be perfect, but we are the family next door. Whether anyone wants to talk about the elephant in the room or not, I will. I will talk about those that are not the "norm" within our society, because for whatever reason or cause, parents like me and children like my son are the new "norm." The number of children diagnosed with Autism has grown from 1 in 166 when I started writing this book to 1 in 88 children. But regardless of a diagnosis or a label, at the end of the day, they are our children and every single one of them deserves the best education possible because they are our future. Their education, independence and success depends on the tools we give them throughout their lives. I am here to tell our story because we are the new norm, the family next door just like any other, and as I hope to help the family next door to me, I pray one day they will do the same. Wouldn't it be fantastic to live in a world where we all helped one another for the betterment of our kids and our fellow neighbors, not just for ourselves? The elephant in the room is diversity and the appreciation of the diversity that lies within every one of us. It will make our children better C.E.O.'s, doctors, lawyers, politicians, or whatever occupation they hold in the future because they understand the most important value a person can have: compassion.

At the age of nineteen, I put myself through a small yet prestigious university by stewardessing on private mega-yachts. Every single holiday and summer I crewed for some of the wealthiest families in the country: socialites, Hollywood movie stars as well as high profile corporate business men and women, from Steven Spielberg, Clint Eastwood, Steven Ross of Time Warner, Jerry Jones of the Dallas Cowboys to the Coca Cola and Pepsi heiresses. At twenty-two, I was lucky enough to work for a gentleman by the name of Henry Mellon of the Mellon banking fortune as his executive assistant for almost four years. I was tireless, and those like the Mellon family not only saw and appreciated my efforts, but also gave me my first career breaks which I will never forget. They also gave me the very beginning foundations for compassion and respect for philanthropy in order to better the lives of others, without wanting or needing anything in return. When I was twenty-three years old, I started my first company designing mega-yachts, traveling around the world in private and corporate jets, dining with society's elite and working seven days a week, often sixteen to seventeen hours a day to be the best that I could and reap the financial rewards. These were days I will never forget, yet the one thing I can honestly say after all these years is they never completed me as a person, nor did they define me.

My calling to help those that have mobility issues, neurological disorders, intellectual disabilities or even the parent who just needs a shoulder to cry on or voice to be heard resonates within every fiber of my being. It's not about how much money I've made or what I have purchased or who I know or have known in life. It's about what I did or will do to improve someone else's life, even if it were for just one person or child. I want to leave this earth knowing I lived and cared for others to the best of my ability regardless of my own self interests. I want and will help others in need because it is the right thing to do for the good of all humanity. Letting go of those who didn't empower me and the materialstic things that just occupied my time and space allowed me to be the person I always wanted to be. I will be the change I want to see in the world because I truly know, even as one person, I can.

As I scan the news and reality television shows, it has become more and more apparent just how much a new social paradigm is needed, a country where we stop looking at the color of one's skin or the car in their driveway or the home they live in. We must look at one another to empower each other and to make each other's lives just a little easier to live. It can begin with something as simple as opening a door for someone at the post office or grocery store, or allowing a car to merge onto the highway though it may delay you for a few seconds, or perhaps even allowing a child—any child—to enter his or her classroom and be welcomed regardless of their ability level, or lack thereof. It takes so much less energy to smile, accept and be kind to one another than to argue, fight, shun, bully or ostracize. We can change the course of our lives by just believing and never giving up.

As I finish my Masters Degree in Early Childhood Special Education and apply for my Ph.D. in Community Leadership and Policy Studies at the University of Vermont, I am reminded of all of those that have helped Taylor and me get to where we are today. The outreach may not have been massive or from the people I would have thought, but I remember every single person that did reach out and help, even in the slightest way. Without them, I never would have had the courage to keep forging ahead and to help pass this compassion on to others: from my Florida family, to my best girlfriends, my best friend, Gavin, my father and second mother, the most amazing people at the University of Vermont, and most definitely my son.

I am proud to say my greatest accomplishment is my son Taylor. Twenty years ago, I couldn't have imagined having a child with special needs, and yet, I have to laugh, as he seems to be the normal one; I on the other hand seem to feel like the odd duck constantly trying to fit into his life. His overwhelming happiness, joy and infectious laugh show me what IS possible rather than what isn't, and how much love and kindness a human being can give to others regardless of an intellectual disabilty.

Reflecting back on those that I admire and those who are helping to address important issues, a very special researcher, Dr. William Mobley, comes to mind for what he has done as a scientist and what he continues to do in pursuit of cognitive improvement for those within the Down syndrome community as well people suffering from Alzheimers. I had been tracking Dr. Mobley's research and findings since my son's birth almost eight years ago when he was the Director of the Center for Research and Treatment of Down syndrome at Stanford University. The labratory under Dr. Mobley made extrodinary progress in tracking the signaling biology of neurotrophic factors in the normal brain and in animal models of neurodegenerative disorders, such as Alzheimer's disease and Down syndrome. He moved on to the University of California at San Diego in June of 2009 to the Center for Neural Circuits and Behavior, where his work continues in the pursuit of helping people with Down syndrome as well as understanding the relationship of Down syndrome and Alzheimers. As I continue to be one of his biggest fans, I remain relentless in supporting all of his efforts as well as everyone working so hard within his laboratory.

It is my time now to rise to the occasion, push myself beyond my comfort zone and be the best I can be, and I hope to encourage others to do the same, because we are all part of this moment in time. We need to talk about the elephants in the room and support each other now more than ever. As I continue to fight and advocate for people with disabilities, I strongly urge everyone to look within his or her own community to find ways to better the lives of others. Support taxes for education, and the proper implementation of these taxes by legislators for all children; support better salaries for teachers, educational therapists and classroom paraprofessionals. Supporting our children's education and well being not only helps their future, but ours as well. We must teach our children how it might feel if they were bullied, teased or shunned at school or within their community, and talk about how they can help stop the negativity before it starts. We must give our children the power of their own voice and affirm the importance of helping and respecting one another. But this begins with you. The next time you see someone with a neurolgical disorder, intellectual disability or mobility issue think how would it feel if the shoe were on the other foot? Think of how you would want others to treat or help you where you needed it. What tools would you need to access your education, community or build life skills if you did have a disability? Think, act, and help those around you for the greater good of humanity not because we expect a return, but because it is the right thing to do. We can create a better world if we just believe, trust, respect, help and support one another.

In looking at the years ahead, I do see promise, hope and the possibility of a new paradigm of thought if we just believe, never give up and work hard for a better tomorrow. Sometimes it just starts with one person and a really, really big dream.

CHAPTER 1

Adversity

A s I lay on the bleach-faded sheets of my hospital bed, a nurse helped to put a surgical cap over my head, gently tucking my long blonde hair under the elastic band. She spoke with calm and ease, assuring me everything was going to be okay. Step by step, she began explaining the events that were about to follow. My baby was in trouble and they needed to perform an emergency c-section. He wasn't getting enough oxygen and his heart rate was dropping drastically.

The memories of the night before kept coming back to me. I could feel him kicking within and then nothing for several seconds. Then a kick, then nothing. My husband and I were having what I was hoping would be, a nice quiet dinner in anticipation of our son. As my husband poured glass after glass of wine before dinner, I asked him to hold back in case I went into labor and he needed to drive me to the hospital. The day before, my doctor had tried to induce labor, given that the baby was overdue. As the evening wore on, I had a mother's instinct that Taylor was ready.

Our feelings of anxiety and anticipation were adding to the tension and unease between us. I kept re-living the events of the past eleven months and in spite of them I was still trying to build my imaginary white picket fence and find normalcy in our relationship. My strength and courage would bring me through everything, I thought; it was my duty as a wife, after all, and the duty of a mother-to-be. It was my job, my calling to fix everything that was wrong with our relatively new marriage, but another part of me also knew that pride simply wouldn't let me

1

show the outside world our dysfunction. I knew I had made a mistake in marrying him.

After nine months, I desperately wanted a calm and inviting home, and I wanted everyone to feel the excitement. Before I knew it though, my request had escalated into yet another argument. I was afraid of a child being born into this environment. Regardless of what I did or what I said, I lived in the shadow of his next confrontation.

Now, at the final hour, I had completely run out of energy and the last thing I wanted to do was argue with someone. I just wanted my imaginary *Town and Country* magazine home to be, somehow, magically real—a life mirroring all of my years of self-education, hard work, my capacity to love and care for people and an insatiable desire to live life to the fullest with my dreamed soul mate.

But he was not my soul mate. He seemed to curb his insecurities with a wine bottle and guitar. His drinking was life itself. The closeness of the wine country was a constant temptation as well as his justification for another wine tasting. He felt it was a part of his cultivation of new business alliances and clients in real estate as well as the link between him and his friends. A few bottles always sat in the corner of the kitchen loosely corked, just waiting for their devilish unveiling night after night. With each pour, his hidden anger would surface.

The night before our son was to be born was no different. As he drank and ignored my request for moderation I felt the need for a hot bath and the warmth and comfort of my fluffy down pillows and down comforter. I could hear the guitar stemming away at his finger tips as I slipped into an exhausted sleep. I tried to move back to my Zen mode of thought and not let the dysfunction outweigh my excitement for my child.

Just as so many nights before, he continued to drink as I slept. In his usual pattern he would wake me from a dead sleep "to ask me a question" in his aggravated and oddly aggressive voice. As the words bounced off the bedroom walls, I winced at the thought of yet another night of no sleep and the possibility of more physical and mental harm. Rather than battle, I picked up a pillow, headed to the linen closet for a warm blanket and regressed back downstairs to sleep on the sofa. It was just easier to ignore him and find a safe hole to crawl in.

After hours of lying on the sofa trying to get comfortable, I hoped this was the night I would meet my child. Over the past nine months, the anticipation was all I could hold on to. It became easier and easier to block out anything negative around me to prepare for his birth. This was my dream and I couldn't wait to see his tiny little face.

Around 11 PM some slight cramping in my belly began. And then throughout the night, more intense cramping followed by the baby's slight movements. By around 5 AM, I knew something just wasn't right. My baby and I had a language of unspoken words. Within an hour and a half, I would be laying on a surgical bed worrying about his survival.

I called my mother around 5:15 AM in Southern California to ask her advice and describe what I was feeling. "Mom, something isn't right. I keep feeling hard cramps like a menstrual cycle and then there is just silence and nothing at all."

"Kimberly, you need to call the doctor and get his advice. I can be on the next plane to meet you at the hospital." I called the doctor immediately, and after discussing everything I had been feeling, he insisted I go to the emergency room as soon as possible.

I knocked on the master bedroom door with enough grace to not wake him with a jolt. I didn't need more problems, just a ride to the hospital. After I explained what was happening, he opened the door. The entire room smelled of stale wine. He dressed and sauntered downstairs to make coffee. I knew better than to push him too much, especially after his actions the night before. So, with a gentle persuasion I said, "I really think I should leave for the hospital now. The baby just doesn't feel right". He pulled the to-go cup from the cabinet, loaded it up with hot coffee, and we left. As we reached the garage, I noticed the almost flat tire on my VW wagon still hadn't been repaired after weeks of asking him to fix it. So, as I sat in the car in labor with a possibly distressed unborn child, we stopped at the local gas station along the way to fill it. I just wanted to scream, "Wake up! You are 48 years old! You need to care for your wife and soon-to-be newborn son!"

After we arrived, the room began to flood with a flurry of hurried doctors and nurses, though it seemed as if everyone were in a regular routine; this was just another part of their daily schedule. But to me, this was completely unchartered territory. My mind began racing and I was desperately trying not to panic. An I.V. stuck painfully out of my left hand, and all I wanted to do was rip it out. The doctor had been in such a hurry to get me into the operating room, he had jabbed it in himself not waiting for the nurse to find my vein. I was so afraid I would feel the same excruciating pain of the initial jab, I didn't say anything. I just wanted a baby. A healthy, happy, beautiful little boy. I could never have imagined in my wildest nightmares any of this would happen as I lay on the hospital bed waiting for reason.

For what seemed like an eternity, I laid in silence watching the nurses getting the room and me ready. The smell of the sterilizing alcohol was making me nauseous. It was so clean, so cold. The bright fluorescent lights hung over my head with a large circular magnifying lamp. It slowly began to dawn on me. *My baby was in trouble and this was an emergency c-section. I was in an operating room.* The nurse calmly explained that I needed an epidural and it would be injected into my spine. It was very, very important that I listen very carefully and do exactly as they instructed. I remember hearing stories about this: What would happen to my baby if I moved at all? Would he feel this large needle as well? The nurse gently explained I needed to very carefully sit up with my legs over the edge of the bed so they could administer the shot. It was so freezing cold and the stiff white sheet and thin woven cotton blanket wasn't enough. And this I.V. in my hand. It was really bothering me now. I became fixated on the simplest things. *The shot—focus. I need to focus on the shot.*

My mind raced back to my Lamaze class. The living room. *Remember the living room.* If anything should ever go wrong, something unexpected during my delivery, the Lamaze instructor said to picture yourself in your place of calm in your mind. Pretend you are in your living room in complete calm. So, I moved my mind and complete focus into my living room. The entire operating room seemed to calm down. It was quieter and for a few brief seconds I found pockets of silence and a renewed hope that all would be fine. The lights were still obnoxiously bright, and people were still hurried, and it was still freezing cold, but then I remembered my baby. I was moving into the zone deep in my mind, just as I had found the same zone I was trained to focus with while racing the high banks of Daytona Motor Speedway. My mind flashed back remembering the rush of adrenaline pumping through my veins as I approached each concrete barrier at 180 miles per hour. Packs of almost thirty other motorcycle racers battling for placement ahead of one another at almost 200 miles per hour on the straights of the track. If I made one false move, I would crash into a concrete wall or worse. I remembered approaching certain turns at Daytona's track where I found myself not breathing, with the G-force in the high outer banks of the track so strong I felt my eyes would explode from the pressure. Yet, as I approached the stands of thousands watching the race, I was able to re-focus and the only thing I would hear was my breath against my helmet's visor and the calm of the zone within my mind. The feeling was euphoric in its simplicity and unlike anything I had ever felt or experienced before as time seemed to stop, and I found an inner peace and calm of the present moment. After so many years of racing and training, I was conditioned to not only lead, but also to focus in life and death situations. Just as had I reached the zone in my mind of calm to process the intensity of the sport, I knew once again, I could certainly reach the same zone of calm, peace and awareness to bring this child into the world safely. My baby needed me to focus and breathe without panic, now more than ever.

Breathe. If I stayed calm, and everyone else in the room focused just the same, my baby would feel the same warmth and welcome into the world. I quickly moved the focus to calming him down. My mind tried to reach his. *Baby, I'm here, and everything is going to be fine. You are fine angel, just stay with me and I promise everything is going to be okay; we are all here for you, and we will help you.* I kept looking for someone to be there for me but there wasn't. Just a room full of strangers and a man that was supposed to be my husband, yet I never felt further from a person in my life. He was a complete stranger that seemed to be observing rather than participating. There was no hand holding; he had turned into a cold shadow, a grimace on his face. It was over between him and me. His malicious and perverse intentions to control and dominate me for the past eleven months became apparent and I saw him for the first time as he was, rather than who I envisioned him to be. He stood in the hospital room for some fake social grace, to report back to his clients, friends and ex-girlfriend, but by no means was he a part of my child's birth as a father. A future dead beat dad that would never be a decent, loving, nurturing mentor for my son. With the birth of a child, it all came to a screeching halt.

The nurse at my side slowly lifted me and helped to swing my legs to the left over the edge of the bed. My gown was coming undone in the back and the I.V. still jabbed into me. *Calm. Go back to calm.* "There will be a small prick of a needle just slightly to the left of your spine, just north of your left butt cheek," the nurse explained "and this will numb the area for the epidural." A few minutes later, with her reassuring arm around my shoulders, she asked me not to move as they were going to administer the large needle. Back to the peace and calm of my imaginary living room. *Baby—don't worry—I'm here.* All I could think of was my baby being okay as a small team slowly laid me back down on the table. The doctor seemed agitated. It was going too slowly for the baby—he needed to begin the c-section. A large blue cloth was flagged over my waist and I could no longer feel my legs. There were suddenly so many people in the room all below the blue cloth, and perhaps the nurse noticed and felt my growing anticipation as she began to stroke my forehead just as my grandmother had done when I was a little girl. This was now the new focus, and it was comforting to know even if she was a stranger, she was at least there for me. It was incredibly calming and felt so good in the chaos of the room, and a relief to know someone seemed to care about me, my baby and our personal well being.

I had never been an overly religious person, however, for the first time in my life, I truly felt the presence of God by my side and He seemed to blanket my child and I with an unexplained sheltering feeling of love, support and safety.

The nurse moved to the doctor's side to help with the delivery, leaving me without a companion. Why is this happening? What is wrong with my child? I wished someone could just tell me step by step what they were doing down there, but then at the same time, perhaps I didn't want to know. I didn't want too many details—just a baby boy healthy and safe. I had a numb feeling as the doctor manipulated my belly and its organs. No one ever explained the process of a c-section to me, and I never inquired because I never in a million years imagined I would be in this room freezing cold . . . and seemingly alone. My mother had been called and she was on the next flight up from Southern California. But where was she?

For nine months of anticipation and planning, I remained ecstatic to meet this little boy. It all seemed so incredibly surreal. And then, just as my doctor finished telling the details of what he was doing for the upcoming weekend, they announced my son was out. A gentle baby's cry. Just beyond the top of the blue sheet, I could barely see a tiny red baby. They asked my husband if he wanted to cut the cord. With a nod yes, he was handed the scissors. Within a minute or so, there were slight hushed tones. The entire atmosphere of the room died down, to a quiet lull from the excitement that had filled it for what seemed like hours. I was waiting for the congratulations and cheers, but the room instead became quiet. I forgot the I.V., the stiff sheets and the room's coldness. The lights seemed to dim again. The nurses gently cleaned, weighed him, and then swaddled my new little bundle of joy tightly in a blue blanket with a powder blue print on it. As they lay him on my chest, his tongue was slightly out between his tiny little lips. His eyes were closed, but I noticed they were slanted.

Why do you have these tiny little features? He was different from any baby I had ever seen before. In a wave of emotions, I said gently enough for only him to hear, "It doesn't matter handsome, we are in this together and whatever it is we will figure it out together." Welcome, Taylor! You are so beautiful!

The hushed tones were now gone in the sterile white room of half masked nurses and doctors. I had heard them, and their label for my son. And yet I didn't care. He was my beautiful little boy. *Whatever it is baby, we'll figure it out.* A male nurse had said Down syndrome. No, no, the others hushed. It felt like a tornado was slowly churning in my room. The words were swirling, the hushes were gathering, and still I was waiting for an I love you . . . a kiss . . . I knew from that moment on I was alone and yet, I wasn't. A part of me was finally complete because I was now a mother. Yet the overwhelming feeling of loneliness kept engulfing me. I felt one with my child. It was the crowd of people around me who made me feel lonely. Who cares if there is something different about him? He is a beautiful and amazing gift. The nurse reached for him to make sure everything was okay and check all of his vitals, and with a swift motion he was gone from my arms, and all I could think of was having him back.

I awoke to complete silence. I was completely alone in a freezing cold stark white room with the smell of oxidized hospital sheets. Where was everyone and where was my son? My husband had been there, even if in the far distance, but now I was on a gurney behind a drawn hospital drape. As I gathered my thoughts, I tried to pull my legs over the edge of the gurney. It was impossible. I was paralyzed. Just as a wave of panic began, a nurse appeared at my side. She said my son was fine, and he was just down the hall with my mother and husband. I was in the recovery room, and I would be taken to my room as soon as the anesthesia wore off. It all came back to me. My son, Taylor.

I had a new friend. A new beautiful son. I couldn't wait to see him again; I just needed to get out of this bed. I couldn't wait to see that precious little face again.

An hour or so later, I was brought to my room and was able to hold Taylor for a little while. He was so sweet, so tiny. For a few minutes my mother, my husband, and I were in the room together, finally celebrating this beautiful little boy. We were in a short grace period; nothing was wrong with my marriage or my perfect child. He was just the most precious little boy I had ever seen with a ton of blond hair with the tiniest little fingers and toes. Perfect little hands and feet that looked like delicate little champagne grapes—the most angelic and magnificent baby I had ever envisioned. I never thought this day would come. He was only five pounds four ounces. So, so tiny with some quirky little facial features. Ever so slight. The more I mulled this over in the depths of my mind, I realized it didn't matter. I was finally a mom after all of the years of anticipation. Overwhelming feelings of gratefulness and honor kept engulfing me. A nurse came to gather Taylor once again and said I needed my rest, and Taylor needed to be looked over again. I kissed Taylor and promised I'd see him as soon as possible.

In the midst of doctors and nurses coming and going in and out of my room, a woman appeared in a casual suit with a small leather bound notebook. Reaching out for my spouse's hand to shake and then mine, she graciously introduced herself, "Hi, I'm Marjorie." She began asking how we were doing and how I in particular was holding up. My husband was still in a daze from the night before, and all of the events leading up to this moment. We were both in a grey fog. I couldn't figure out why she was there. The pain medication had made me woozy and unable to focus. After his prodding of who she was and why she was here, she announced she was from social services and was following up on my case. Her timing could not have been any worse. The glare in his eyes left chills down my spine. He quickly thanked her for stopping by, but adamantly insisted everything was fine; we would call her if we needed her.

My mind flashed backed to a room similar to this one, with a police officer by my side. He was asking me how the fall happened as we together glanced down at the baby monitors hooked up to my belly. I was explaining to him how I was thrown to the ground two times by my husband as I was trying to flee my home and him. He had been in another rage and was dragging me back into the kitchen as I was on the ground, seven months pregnant.

The flashback faded as I then realized this woman had my medical file and she was checking to make sure I was okay, which I could only assume was a precaution when domestic violence of a pregnant woman is charted in a file. She left the room, and the moment the door was closed he went into the angry rant I had grown accustomed to. He blamed me for her presence and visit, as if somehow I asked her to come. Then, just as abruptly, he sat on the edge of my bed sobbing. He clearly was not going to be strong enough to cope with what lay ahead. And I knew I not only was on my own, but now that the baby was born, I had to be on my own for the child's sake. Once again, I was consoling him, to downgrade the anger and other emotions that usually followed this behavior; it was easier than fighting it.

As I lay in my bed, I kept going back to the happy places in my mind, thinking of the next day or the following when Taylor could come home. My strength came from creating the little white picket fence in my mind I had always dreamed of, a trick I had used since I was a little girl to shelter my mind from the pain of the dysfunction that surrounded me. It was how I survived the hard times and created a sense of peace and calm in my mind until I figured out how to make things better.

I had spent months researching the clothing he would need, the diapers, the colorful geometric mobile for over his crib. It was a perfect baby's room when I finished with it. My family and friends had sent so many amazing gifts of clothing, toys and decorations all befitting a little boy and I used every single piece to make it all look perfect down to the very last detail. The clothing was neatly arranged on little white silk padded hangers in his closet and color coded as well as his socks that were meticulously organized and put away. To have a child was an amazing gift and I wanted to savor every moment of the process.

I will figure out the problems with my husband and me. I was a fixer, and I could fix this. Or could I? Failure was never an option, and I was determined not to fail at beginning a new family. Perhaps though, the original family model I anticipated wouldn't be the same as the one we actually lived in our every day. My hopes had begun to unravel eleven months before, the first time he raised his voice to me and threw me up against a wall. I just didn't have the strength at the time to call it off, and certainly not after I was carrying a child. Perhaps the worst part of our relationship were the cover-ups for family and friends. Swallowing my pride and confessing to my friends and family I had made one of the gravest mistakes in my life by marrying the wrong man was just too great of a task for me to bear.

After I had slept a little longer, the head nurse and attending doctor came into the room to talk. The doctor said Taylor was having difficulties breathing. Evidently, the umbilical cord was short, and bradycardia, or slow heart rate was detected. There was a slight heart murmur, he was jaundiced and needed more in depth NICU care than they could provide. As the doctor was explaining the details, Taylor was already being prepped for ambulatory movement to the University of San Francisco Pediatric Hospital and was to be transported within hours. My mind was swirling with fear and questions. I knew they had put a label on him that I still didn't understand, but I never expected anything more. He was just in my room, in my arms, and he seemed fine. I began bracing myself and moving back into the zone of my mind from my conditioning and athletic training in order to regain the strength I was going to need to get through whatever lay ahead.

We saw Taylor in the hallway around 5 PM as they were getting ready to transport him in a large red incubator, with monitoring wires lacing his tiny body and oxygen tubes in his nose. As I stared at the huge machine with this tiny little baby inside, I couldn't believe it was happening. I had done everything during my pregnancy to make sure the baby would be healthy: organic, healthy foods, lots of exercise, but there was never a sign anything close to this would happen. I said my goodbyes as the two paramedics wheeled the huge machine away with my tiny baby in it. My breath came ragged, and shallow, time seemed to stop. The room and sounds around me seemed to fall into complete silence. I didn't hear any one or see any one and it felt as if my body were completely numb. I just wanted to hold him and take him home. I was alone again. I could feel my husband begin to stir uneasily as we reached the confines of my hospital room. The gesture of spending the night with me in light of our change in circumstances and grief was never offered. He would be off to drink again.

My mother had an art show back in Southern California, and had gone the night before, and my husband had left after dinner the night before. He had insisted we not tell anyone of the label the doctor and nurses were giving Taylor until the test results were in. I went to sleep alone that night and awoke alone, when all I wanted to do was hold my newborn son and be embraced by a husband that had now become a complete stranger, and perhaps always was. The next morning I spoke to the nurse regarding my release. They needed to evaluate me and the doctor needed to sign a release form. By 9:30 my husband was still at home having coffee and the doctor still hadn't come to my room. Patience worn thin, I got dressed and prepared myself to take a cab the twenty-two miles into the city to get to Taylor. No absentee husband or doctor's signature would stop me.

The drive across the bridge was surreal. The sky was a clear and cloudless California blue, and the Sienna hills framed the bridge's span as if to say, with open arms, you're almost there. I arrived at the University of California San Francisco Moffit Hospital around 11 a.m. on a brisk but beautifully sunny San Francisco day. As I made the long trek through the hospital and all of the security check points for the NICU section of the hospital, I realized just how serious the course of events had become. I was realizing just how ill my son was, and I knew I needed to get to him and help him. Finally reaching the room and meeting his head nurse, I heaved a huge sigh of relief. His bed was in the far corner by the window with a rocking chair beside it and the view just outside the window beside his crib was spectacular, overlooking Golden Gate Park and the botanical gardens. Our nurse instructed me to thoroughly scrub my hands up to my elbows with a brush and to remember to do this every time I entered the room. The smell of the soap still lingers in my mind, as does the feeling of the tiny bristles of the brush against my skin. He was wrapped in a blanket in his tiny little bed, with the cutest little pink and blue striped knit cap and shades over his eyes to protect them from the incubator lights. He looked like he was at the beach.

I was given the full tour and all of the instructions for Taylor's day-to-day care with every aspect and detail; it all seemed incredibly compartmentalized and intricate. We had to weigh his diapers every few hours and all of his vitals were constantly being monitored. Everything was carefully and meticulously charted: from his oxygen levels by a clamp on his finger, to the EKG monitor. Hour after hour, every day I helped nurse him back to health. Ten to twelve hours every day I just sat and stared at this beautiful little boy praying he would live. The care of his team was the most extraordinary experience I have ever known and the nurses gave me the strength and confidence to keep my own personal strength.

Every morning and every evening it was an incredible feat to get Taylor's father to visit. He seemed incapable of compassion and unwilling to take up the responsibilities of our new life, and I had watched the patterns for nine months as his son's birth grew near. I hadn't wanted to believe it, nor could I tell my family it wasn't going to work out between us for myself, and now more importantly for my child. I would leave Taylor for a half hour, only to eat lunch alone in the hospital cafeteria, wondering how many other families were going through this same situation. I wished I knew who they were; I wished I could talk to someone. I was developing a plan B with every lonely day I was spending sitting next to this beautiful child fighting for his life day in and day out. He deserved more than a man who couldn't bother to be there at such a critical time in our lives. Day after day as I sat in the NICU, I kept beating myself up for not taking more time, for not paying attention to all of the red flags, and for eventually marrying a man that so reminded me of the many destructive qualities my father had when I was a little girl. Now I was realizing each hour and day that I just had to keep the focus on Taylor and his well being; the rest I assured myself would follow and I prayed often for Taylor and me and for a future of lots of laughter, love and happiness.

The various teams made their rounds in intervals throughout the day. From doctors to students, all discussing the conditions and needs of all of the children. It was fantastic to see such intense training for the students, and the nurses couldn't have been any more professional or kind. I felt safe there and almost wished the days wouldn't end, because they surrounded Taylor and I like a family, doting over everything my son needed with precision. In the whirlwind of all of the events leading up to Taylor's birth, that simple room overlooking the lush green grounds of Golden Gate Park was our newfound home of safety, warmth and love felt by everyone that was a part of it or passed through it. The experience at UCSF's (University of San Francisco Children's Hospital), NICU will forever be a defining moment in my life, as it taught me a new level of care giving and compassion demonstrated by each and every staff member. They gave me hope of what was possible after almost loosing my baby to a series of medical complications. Each and every doctor, nurse and team member were a resource and comfort in a community setting making me hope and pray to find one just like it outside the hospital walls.

A culture was taken to determine Taylor's prognosis. Maybe it wasn't Down syndrome. Or maybe it was only a Mosaic or—"lesser" form of Down syndrome. I kept asking myself—why is this so important? Who cares? So my son has some issues. The only important issue was getting Taylor to breathe without an oxygen tube, and eat on his own. This is what is really important. On the sixth day the doctor handed us a funny sheet with squiggles all over it. Taylor was born with forty-seven chromosomes with an extra twenty-first. He had Down syndrome. Okay. Now that that part is over—do we still need to discuss this I thought? I just wanted to celebrate the birth of a child, and now there was this enormous black shadow everyone was casting on it. This huge label.

My husband was devastated and crying. At night, after I had spent the long day at the hospital, his drinking became worse and so did his denial of Taylor's diagnosis. He just didn't want to talk about it. I found myself comforting everyone else. There was no time to grieve. I was caring for Taylor all day and then my husband by night.

The same day we were told Taylor's diagnosis, I made it a priority to visit the hospital library where I found medical books in which we could reference Down syndrome, and understand what it was. They described all of the complications and various physical and mental health issues that might occur, but they didn't have any reading material about what all these children would and could do; it was all completely negative, feeding feelings of devastation instead of celebration. In the back of my mind I found this so bizarre. Would he never speak, walk, eat on his own? All we found were medical journals filled with medical terms and a horrible label of mental retardation. The words rattled like an earthquake every time I heard it. How can this be? Why? And how did it happen? Was it my fault?

Finally, on the eighth day, Taylor was breathing on his own, and breast feeding well enough to be released. He did have a small hole in his heart valve that might not close over time. Surgery was a possibility later, but it was small enough not to be of significant concern right then. His jaundice was gone, and he showed no other signs for concern. Still, I was beyond terrified on so many levels. The known was this room where everyone cared for Taylor and me. I was told what to do in great detail for when we were home, however he didn't come with an instruction manual, and

I really felt like I needed one. Now we were both being released into the world with a label that I had no idea what it really meant and a husband unable to cope. I kept thinking there should be a nurse to help me. He's just too tiny. I can't do this. I'm not strong enough to handle all of this. Then, just as quickly as he had arrived, Taylor was carefully strapped into the back seat and away we went. My work was just about to begin and so was our new life.

CHAPTER 2

Freedom

The first days of Taylor being home were filled with so many emotional extremes it was difficult to put into words. He was so tiny and quiet, barely ever crying. Terrified to go far from his side, I opted for a small basket for him to sleep in so I could monitor him twenty-four hours a day while he slept next to me. I felt like I still needed to weigh his diapers, chart his feedings, and sterilize everything and everyone that walked in the door; I didn't, but it was hard trusting that everything would be okay with him under my watch and not under a nurse or doctor's care.

I learned to take everything hour by hour, eventually working towards day by day. We slowly began to tell our friends and family that Taylor had Down syndrome, although it would take weeks to really talk about it and years to accept and understand what it really meant. The first weeks however didn't so much amplify the diagnosis itself, but what it meant to others. To me, it was my son Taylor, and that was all. He happened to have a label too, but it didn't define him. Sadly, there weren't enough people that could fathom this. My mother was completely supportive and generous with her time, flying back and forth from Southern California to San Francisco to help. Despite the tensions within our home, she persevered, however, not without great consequences to me. My husband and mother were both having trouble processing the label that followed my son, and their grief, whether they realized it or not, was completely self-absorbing. They had to bear their pain and grief on their own. I couldn't have anything to do with it, for the mere fact I needed to keep my strength to recover from a c-section and care for my son. Dwelling on what they perceived as a loss in not having a typical child only resulted in an even greater need for control over the situation, over Taylor and over me. I was now being told what to do, how to act, with whom I was and was not to communicate with. My life was no longer mine but completely theirs. Everyone deals with life's challenges differently, however Taylor's label became an impetus for me to do something I never imagined: let go of my own ego and self-absorption. It was no longer about me, my faults, my insecurities, my fears, my sadness. It was about my son and whatever support he needed to live a happy, healthy and valued life. My own self doubts only led to fear the unknowns of having a child with extra needs, instead of just allowing myself to accept things as they stood. I had to work on letting go of the expectations of what my life was supposed to look like and start focusing on what I now wanted for my son's happiness and success.

The people who stared at Taylor with unwelcoming eyes seemed to always be those who were afraid to face their own issues of adversity. It's taken me a long time since Taylor's birth to understand it without having anger towards them. Day after day as he grows older, walking through the grocery store or at the park, I see and feel the stares, the comments, and often wonder how they would feel if they were standing in my shoes and if they would think differently under the same circumstances. Or was I truly an anomaly? I prayed every day for people to look beyond the differences.

And so, as we talked to our friends and family, I began to confide in those I could trust to have no judgment and who were just as happy as I that Taylor was finally here. I clung to my girlfriends' every word of support and love, and they became my lifeline. They didn't have a personal agenda, they were my friends who just wanted to listen and lend a shoulder to cry on when I needed it. I think the most important dimension in my genuine, close relationships with friends during this period of time was that regardless of what mistakes I was making or what mistakes I had made, especially in my new marriage, they never judged me or left my side. There were many others however who gave up and even blacklisted me within their exclusive social circles. I was ostracized in many regards because I was the one who was in the relationship of domestic violence, instead of understanding I was the one being abused, controlled and manipulated. Somehow the burden was all mine as a woman and I was forced into a society of being the accuser rather than the victim. At the same time, they were still cordial when seeing the man who was the perpetrator at wine tastings, on the ski slopes and at dinner parties. For many years after we divorced, I was shamed into thinking I was the one at fault. With time and in developing this incredible mother-son relationship, I realized anyone that had left my side, wasn't a person I wanted my son to be around anyway. I had been the one with my tail between my legs, living in constant fear for myself and now my son, cowering at this shadow of a man that seemed to never go away in my sub-conscious.

Once Taylor was home, I could no longer hide behind the white picket fence and the many delusions to which I had tried to cling. Everyone asks why I didn't leave, why I waited so long and how it came about that I even married this man. The burden of blame became solely my own according to the outside world. To me, just as I had been conditioned to believe in my childhood, it had to be something I was doing wrong. I began asking myself what in the world had brought me to this particular point in my life and why did I choose such a difficult path? My son became a mirror of what my own childhood looked like, and how tragic many of its elements were as a little girl. I couldn't bear to see a child live through so many of the same pains, especially a child with special needs. I felt I needed to break the chain of dysfunction and violence that I had always known and create a world of peace, calm, happiness and stability for both of us.

My fondest and furthest memory brings me to the tiny town on the East Coast where I was born. My crib at the base of my grandmother's bed was positioned perfectly in front of her single glass-paned picture window with the most beautiful white church steeple in the distance. At night, I would rise onto my toes to see over the crib's railing and gaze at the dazzling white lights outlining the high pitched steeple. I had some strange calling every time I spent the night at my grandmother's to stare as long as I could, to feel the peace of its presence. Maybe it was the steeple and bright lights for a young child, or maybe it was something much deeper, more spiritual, that drew me in like a magnet.

Even at this early age, I craved attention and affection from where ever I could get it. My grandmother was always there for me with her eyes like blue topaz and ever so long, romantic stories of how she and my grandfather had first met on the shores of Lake George in New York. We would sit for hours and talk about the happiest times of the 1940's and 1950's, of her childhood and early teenage years, and her first years as a secretary in Washington D.C. I gratefully spent a lot of time with my grandmother and grandfather as year after year it became a reprieve from the denial, anger and dysfunction within my parent's home.

My mother and father met in their small town on the East Coast, dated throughout high school and eventually married in their early 20's. He bought his first home in a neighboring town where they welcomed a baby boy, and then almost three years later, a little tow headed blonde appeared, me. My father always dreamed of California and becoming an architect, so, when I was six months old, he took the leap, sold our small town home and moved to California to pursue his lifelong dream. We spent the next nine years moving from apartment to apartment, home to home between Reno, Nevada and the Bay Area of San Francisco. The pressures of college and raising two children at the ripe age of twenty-five brought many hurdles and challenges for both of them.

Over the course of my first nine years of life, my mother, brother and I moved back to the East Coast several times, only to end back again with my father. It wouldn't have been that bad I suppose if my father didn't have such pent up anger and hostility. They argued behind closed doors so my brother and I didn't hear as much of it; I'm still trying to figure out if that was a good thing. The inability to grasp onto an argument or locate a cause of his anger somehow made it even more confusing as children. As an adult I look back, and consciously know it wasn't us at all. He was a man incredibly unhappy with himself and his circumstances at a period in his life when he wasn't able to manage as a father or husband. My brother and I were just innocent outlets.

In the presence of their friends and at our own dinner table, we were always taught to not speak unless spoken to, and never, ever speak with an opinion while he was speaking, or while he was watching television. The golden rules of a man that worked very hard and was looking for a quiet calm at the end of his day. In the mental snapshots of my childhood, I remember the trips leaving my father but none of the trips coming back to live as a family. I remember being perhaps six years old sitting on the luggage seat of our 350 SL Mercedes convertible with my Snoopy doll, driving across the United States with my mother singing away steering ahead as my brother sat complaining in the front seat. Miles of singing and all I can remember is how grand it felt. We were free. Or maybe it was my mother that was free and her happiness filled our car as she guided her children, state by state, to where she envisioned was the proper place for us to be. Or, perhaps it was for herself.

My most difficult years of the family dysfunction lay behind the walls of yet another dream home my father built in the remote countryside on the East Coast. It was an astronomically big four-story barn he was renovating while we lived in it. He implemented with perfection modern amenities in an original barn that once housed cows and bales of hay. He kept all of the original barn beams, and placed clear story glass panes between them giving a 50' x 60' wall of glass leading out onto the circular deck. With our budget, we had to live in the home during every facet of its re-building—washing our dishes in the tub and going to the bathroom in the woods because our plumbing wasn't finished yet, adding to the family stresses. A dream home that held the memory of my saddest day with him, overshadowing the talent he had or the brilliance of his architectural work.

The years of my father's temper flaring at the drop of a hat always left us walking on pins and needles. If my mother wasn't getting the desired behavior from us, she always deferred to, "Just wait until your father comes home!" It was another reinforcer of negative behavior just as my father calling me stupid and retarded when I didn't understand my homework, instead of being compassionate and helpful with my learning disability of dyslexia. I was a child, like any other, trying to communicate and reach out for help but under the circumstances, I had no idea how.

My darkest moment with him brings back the pain of being dragged across the Mexican tile floor by my pony tail as I screamed at the top of my lungs for my mother to help. It felt like every piece of hair, strand for strand, was being ripped out of my scalp. I was pleading for him to stop and for my mother to help yet, once again, my she did nothing. I was a child and I was completely helpless with no one to rescue me. The stories were worse for my brother, but as an adult, I made it "out"; my brother did not. He now lives in a world of alcohol and pain killers with delusions of a life he never lived, still looking for the acceptance of my father.

Finally, and thankfully, my parents divorced when I was thirteen years old. The decision of where I would live was second to the amount of money that was to be divided amongst the two of them. As I entered junior high, my father moved back to his dream, living full time in California, and moving to the richness of the mountains of Lake Tahoe. I remained with my mother and a brother who was just entering the Marine Corps.

My brother's infrequent trips back home were now filled with his self-proclaimed responsibility of raising his sister. And so, I began to find sanctuary in recreational drugs. They allowed me to enter a world of illusions, of peace and happiness away from the angry home life I endured. Just when I thought I was safe, my wonderfully protective brother would return home to "discipline" with an even greater skill set than before. All of his training was "paying off"—learning the various techniques to hurt people and bring them to their knees in pain without bruising.

My best friend and first boyfriend Christopher was from one of the most old fashioned, respected and wholesome families in town and was forever trying to understand why my mother didn't see what my brother was doing to me and why she didn't put a stop to it.

One afternoon after school, Christopher dropped me off at home. For whatever reason, my brother proceeded to verbally break me down in front of Christopher, grabbing me by the forearm and flinging me into the house. Christopher's eyes looked like a deer caught in the headlights and he cringed in fear for me. "Go Christopher. It's okay. I'm used to it; I can handle it". The last thing I wanted was for Christopher to get involved and possibly hurt because of me. It would have broken me. My last memory of that incident after Christopher left, was being thrown against the corner of the formica kitchen countertop and my temple hitting the edge, knocking me out instantly. The perversion of my brother's violence was that he truly believed that I deserved it.

By fifteen, my behavior was only getting worse, and living in my mother's house was now unbearable for both of us. My father agreed perhaps I should try to come live with him in Lake Tahoe, away from my friends and the troubles I seemed to be getting into on the East Coast. For me, all I could think of was, maybe he really finally wants me in his life and we could start fresh—just the two of us. I could show him how fabulous a daughter I could be, and we would live happily ever after. He was articulate, a fabulous designer; despite his temper, he had qualities that I wanted to emulate. I didn't know why, but I needed and wanted his love and acceptance. His rejection was always more than I could bear.

After my ninth grade year, my mother said her goodbyes with great tears welling in her eyes at Newark airport in New Jersey. As I walked down the long walkway of the terminal, I was relieved and scared at the same time. I thought California might be the change I needed, the change for my father and I and our relationship. Yet, I was also scared to live under the tensions I had always associated with him. Despite reservations, my options were limited; I hopped onto the plane not wanting to ever look back. I didn't want to contemplate what my life wasn't but what it could be.

I would forever be fighting an uphill battle proving myself to my family and to myself because I was conditioned to think I was never good enough. No matter what accomplishments or triumphs, at the end of the day, it wouldn't matter. After all of the years of crying and and just wanting their love and attention, I realized it had nothing to do with me; I would never get the positive reinforcement I needed from them. I was by no means an angel from the age that I could walk and talk, and I was a true fighter if you crossed my path; because I had to be. I was a feisty, independent, tenacious, stubborn child with a mind of her own and yet, as I reflect back on my childhood, they were the ones that were weak, and I most certainly wasn't to hold blame. There is never, ever a place in any home for domestic violence.

CHAPTER 3

Survival

We had met in September, were engaged in November, became pregnant in January, and married in February. There were extreme problems from the beginning, and I knew it, but I was determined I could fix them, and him. It all happened so fast, that I never had time to think clearly or rationally, and the thought of raising a child on my own seemed impossible at the time. Hiding behind my own egocentric insecurities until Taylor was born, I couldn't admit to my family I had made such a terrible mistake. I held on, hoping the relationship would fix itself and that perhaps having a child would help bring love and hope into our home.

I remember the ultimatum he gave me before we were married: if we didn't get married by a certain date, I would never see him again and I would be completely on my own raising a child. The words had plagued my mind for weeks, swirling like a storm cloud in my conscious, and remained even as I stood on the jagged cliff edge of the La Jolla coastline in my wedding dress. I was shaking like a leaf trying to pass it off as goose bumps and shivers from the cold. However, it wasn't cold enough for shivers. I was looking at my mother, silently screaming help me, but as had become our pattern, she looked right through me. If I walked away from this scene I would be alone, pregnant, and shamed in the eyes of my family, once again not living up to the expectations I assumed they held for me.

The worst part of the entire scene was the priest handing me a piece of paper to sign after the ceremony. No one had prepared me for this and this act of signing heightened the reality of what was in motion. Once again, I stepped into the shoes of a frightened little girl looking for direction and once again could only hear the crashing of the surf against the cliff's edge. I was now married to a man I barely knew, bound by a ring choking my pregnant swollen finger with a contract holding me financially tied to this stranger for the rest of my life.

In the first week of Taylor being home, and the events leading up to his birth, I was already becoming a single parent. The distance between my spouse and I not only became greater, but he became more volatile. He lacked the ability to cope; the adversity was just too painful and foreign for him. There was absolutely nothing I could do to save him, let alone our marriage, nor at this point did I want to.

Within three days of Taylor's arrival home, my mother had flown back from Southern California to lend a hand with Taylor while I recuperated. He was twelve days old and doing well with his feedings, sleeping most of the time, and waking every three hours or so. He was an angel and had completely recovered after his initial medical complications. Now, we were just trying to get used to the routine and find a calm balance within our home.

The neighboring town was having a huge Oktoberfest on a perfect fall day, with giant white marshmallow clouds floating over head and in the bright, blue California sky. Still apprehensive about traveling far from Taylor's side, I declined my husband's invitation to go with him and join in the festivities. After several hours of beer swilling with friends, he jovially arrived back at our little townhouse as happy as could be. He was in rare form, loving his little family, even my mother and her presence. As the hours passed, and the beer swilling turned into wine, I began to see his volatile temper crackle under the surface. I felt the angst of what I feared the most. Praying this wouldn't happen in front of my mother, and just four days after Taylor's arrival in his new home; I did everything I could to walk on the egg shells that were all too familiar. I excused myself early from the night, and went to bed. The best way to diffuse the possibility of his antics was to just remove myself. Sure enough, an hour or two later, he awoke me with the usual phrase, "I have a question for you." I'm not sure why this became the hint of the trouble to come, but it always was. Every time he said it, there was sure to be the onslaught of nonsensical behavior and confrontations. Always the exact same phrase after waking me out of a dead sleep.

I was still sore from the surgery and absolutely exhausted, just wanting to sleep any moment I could between Taylor's feedings. "Please let me sleep. We can talk tomorrow," I pleaded gently. Without even having the time to absorb the moment, his lurking rage bubbled over. He was furious I didn't give him the attention or immediate gratification he was looking for. It didn't take much of anything to set him off, and there was nothing I could do that would diffuse this in his demented mind once it started. Nothing. Not getting the reaction he wanted, he stormed out of the room with temples flaring and pounded on the guest bedroom door yelling for my mother to come out and talk. The dreaded moment had come, and my mother was finally going to witness what I had lived in silence and shame over for the past several months. I was mortified, and scared to death at the same time.

He began yelling obscenities, wasn't making any sense and there was certainly no reasoning with him once it got to this point. My mother and I were terrified as the rage within him welled, mostly afraid for the little newborn baby that was only a few feet away sleeping. My son was just home from the NICU, his father was going into a rage and I was his only protection. My husband disappeared downstairs to find the calm in the kitchen of more wine. I lifted Taylor from his crib and swaddled him with a blanket, covering his little ears to shelter him from the tirade that was sure to continue. I quickly pulled him and my mother into the upstairs bathroom and locked the door. It was the only place I could think of on the second floor where the lock actually worked. My mother and I were both shaking, our hearts pounding as we braced ourselves for anything because he sounded so enraged and unpredictable. I had seen him grow this angry a couple of times before, and it was absolutely terrifying.

We stood in the dark of our little bathroom in complete shock. After what seemed like an eternity, he figured out what we had done in locking ourselves in the bathroom, and began banging ferociously on the door. All I could think of was the need to protect my baby and my mother, and there was absolutely no way I would allow this man to harm either of them.

I began to move into survival mode and develop an escape plan. Without a doubt, I would put myself between him and my son and mother to shield them against him. I had no idea what he was capable of, nor was I going to take any chances.

As he realized we weren't budging, the banging on the door stopped, and as he moved back from the door, an eerie, chilling silence followed. I gave it about ten minutes before I opened the door. I sensed he had perhaps gone back downstairs to the safety of the wine bottles. As I opened the door, I instructed my mother to hold Taylor and lock the door behind me, and no matter what she heard, she was not to leave the bathroom with Taylor but stay safely locked behind its wooden barrier.

I carefully walked down the long flight of stairs with my heart racing and breath shallow. As I reached the bottom landing to the stairs, I realized he had grabbed his cell phone, and gone outside; this gave me the seconds I needed to secure my home. As I ran to the back door and locked it, I could hear him talking on the phone in front of our townhouse. I had seen his car keys on the entry table and quickly ran to the front door, grabbing them and removing the house key. With a swift opening of the door, I threw them outside, dead-bolted the door and ran upstairs to get to my mother and Taylor. He realized within minutes what I had done and began screaming obscenities for the entire neighborhood to hear. My shameful little secret was out in the wide open for my mother and everyone else in my community to hear. As we were soon to find out, my wonderful neighbor had called the police on him after hearing his horrific name calling. I could no longer hide behind the mirage of my white picket fence; my dirty little secret of domestic violence was finally out for the world to see and there was definitely no way of turning back.

The police arrived within moments of my neighbor's call, and listened intently to our accounts of the night. Within a half hour, they had woken the judge asking for an emergency restraining order in light of the circumstances, and I was granted a three day order to be enforced by the local police to keep him away. He wasn't going to change, and I now had to protect my child regardless of a fear of him or the fear of what anyone else in the outside world thought about me or the situation. I wasn't going to raise him like this, nor would I ever allow him to know this kind of world ever even existed.

The restraining order left me with three days to pack up my entire home of two and a half bedrooms, antiques, china, clothing, toys, baby crib, everything, and leave. My mother had to go back to Southern California for work, and in the three days that followed her departure, I barely slept, barely ate from nerves, packed, boxed and had a team of movers dismantle everything. My home had looked so perfect with fresh flowers every day, and decorated just as I would have decorated a client's home without a detail unnoticed. Just as my home had been for me as a little girl, no one would ever know the chaos that lived within it because it all looked so aesthetically pleasing and perfect: only smoke and mirrors. I left with Taylor wrapped in my arms and said my goodbyes to my beautiful town house and the chaos that lived within. I would not have anyone treat me the way he had for so long, and there was absolutely no way I was going to allow a child to be a part of such dysfunction. No one deserves to be treated that way, and no man would ever physically or mentally harm me again. Through the birth of a child I had finally found the beauty and strength within me and embraced it with all that I knew I wanted to be not just for myself, but for my son. Taylor gave me the logic, courage and love to respect myself, to say enough is enough and to move on with our lives without such a horrible man. This was the day I realized my son may have in fact just saved my life by his presence and his gift of coming into my life.

I didn't have a lot of time to think about it, but the most practical place to go was Southern California to be closer to my mother, however I had almost no money. I had absolutely no idea how I was going to do this, endlessly thinking night after night, losing more and more sleep in between feedings. Where would the money come from? How would I find the strength? And then, somehow an extra mode of survival kicked in and I went into a state of mind of putting my emotions into actions, just the same as I had racing motorcycles. I didn't think about anything, but instead just forged on and did it.

My father and stepmother had given us a 1947 wooden Chris Craft wooden boat as a wedding gift that was still docked in Lake Tahoe. I knew I could sell the boat for enough money to begin a life with Taylor outside of where we were. It was all I had as a possible liquid asset to support Taylor until I got my feet back on the ground and recuperated physically and mentally. All I could focus on was selling the boat and moving on with the next part of my life as a single mother, and sole provider physically, emotionally and financially for my son.

It sounds ridiculous that the sale of a boat could be so emotionally devastating, but it was. In the midst of this tornado I was in, it was the last real link I felt I had between my father and me. The memories and underlying bond it represented between my father and me was the calm in a whirlwind and now I had to let that go too. We both loved Tahoe and I adored having that one-on-one time with him as an adult. Even though it wasn't a lot of time, it was still ours. He and my step-mother had sold their second home in Tahoe the year before, and decided to stay on the East Coast for their future retirement, leaving the boat behind as a token of their love for me, or perhaps guilt in leaving after I had traveled so far two years prior to be closer to them. I lost my family to 3200 miles away, and now this silly little boat was going too, along with my husband, the white picket fence and the thoughts and hope for a typically developing healthy baby. I again pushed myself to stop thinking too much and put one foot in front of the other. I set my mind to just making it to the end of the day, each and every day. After a few short weeks on the internet, the boat miraculously sold to a wonderful older gentleman in the mid-west that wanted to restore it. It was perfect timing, and the perfect person to care for something that meant so much to me.

I had finished packing everything, put it all into storage until I had a clearer plan and moved to Southern California to be closer to my mother and her support with just a few of Taylor's toys and clothes, all within a few short weeks. I knew no one except for my mother, her husband and a few of her friends from church. I still had an interior design project in Newport, Rhode Island that I was working on which would be my only source of future income, at least in the short term. I also knew there would be a tidal wave of hospital bills for Taylor's stay as well as my surgery, and that this was going to be a complete disaster if I didn't figure everything out as soon as possible. At the same time, I couldn't eat for what seemed weeks, not even a piece of toast. Breast-feeding became impossible as the flow of milk just stopped by six weeks. I was running on adrenaline, but was completely exhausted living in utter survival mode.

Thankfully, as my breast milk had depleted itself to nothing, Taylor transitioned with ease to formula and was doing really, really well. He was a happy, healthy and loving little baby without a care in the world, just as I wanted him to feel. He gave me a renewed energy because I realized at the end of the day, I was all he had and he was the only real, tangible and solid thing I had.

We moved into a tiny, one-bedroom apartment in Southern California overlooking a strip of surfer hangouts and bars. Not ideal, but I was broke and the rent was cheap. We would just have to make the best of it, and it would buy me some time until I figured out something long term. I borrowed some odd pieces of furniture from my mother's house and had a mattress on a frame with Taylor's crib next to me in the bedroom. We had a small T.V. on the floor in the living room and every baby Einstein toy and movie that was out. This was when our Uncle Joe from Florida became incredibly helpful, sending us clothes for Taylor, diapers, toys, and whatever else he could to help me and support Taylor. My mother was also amazing during this period of time, trying to help me adapt me to this strange new town. My best girlfriends continued to talk to me every day from the East Coast, coaching me along through every obstacle, every tear I shed and every fear I had of the unknowns that lay ahead. I was hanging on by a thread, crippled by exhaustion. But, I had a focus: providing the best, most stable, peaceful, loving and safe environment possible for my son. I began reading every book I could find on Down syndrome. I had to help him and give him every resource available regardless of our financial situation; I would find the means.

Shortly after we were settled into our little apartment, I received several phone calls from the district attorney's office from our former Northern California residence, as well as a certified letter requesting my testimony in prosecuting my future ex-husband. They were developing a strong domestic violence case against him with four counts total in jeopardy if I didn't appear and testify against him. I had filed the divorce papers in November of 2004, just seven weeks after my son's birth, and thought I had put the his darkness behind me. I had run, but it was clear I wouldn't be able to hide.

As I fought the custody battle, child support, divorce and now the addition of a possible juried trial, I kept holding on to two words for Taylor and I: survival and freedom. His health, stability and well being were all I cared about and it was my focus at the beginning of each day and at the end of each day. Tenacity was all I had to help him and develop his independence.

In May of 2006, my divorce was final. It took two long years to settle. He signed a release of any visitation or parental involvement in order to not pay child support. By the stroke of a pen, I was now a completely self-supporting single mother. I still remember driving down the highway after leaving my attorney's office just outside San Francisco. Stunned and numb, I realized what this man had just done and how cold and incredibly heart breaking it was as a mother. How could any human being sign off their own child to avoid paying child support? But that was his karma to deal with. Taylor and I were free, safe and I would now see to not only our survival, but also our success in starting a new life.

Of course, despite the joy of now being free to build a life with Taylor, the reality of our situation was a constant fear. I was overwhelmed and severely depressed, finding it difficult even to get up in the morning and put one foot in front of the other after the emotional turmoil. I was alone in a town where I knew five people at the most, with a brand new child and no idea how I would support him; on top of the cost of babysitting, food, rent, diapers. The hardest part was simply leaving the safety of the apartment and this new little boy to go look for a job. I was unable to even think of leaving this little boy I almost lost not so long ago, and terrified to leave him in the hands of another person while I went to some meaningless job.

But it was my new life and I needed to own it, accepting help from my family and friends but not expecting any handouts.

Before I knew it, Christmas came. My mother and I took Taylor to his first Down syndrome group Christmas party at a huge hotel south of the town of Coronado, just below the city of San Diego. Taylor was three months old and the tiniest little boy, resembling a cherub with rosy cheeks, bright blue eyes and white-blond hair. Everyone was having an absolute blast, from teenagers to young children all dancing and laughing. It was like walking into the excitement of Disneyland for the first time. We were complete strangers but everyone greeted us with huge hugs and a feeling of acceptance. Who were all of these people? And why were they so nice?! After all of the battles over the past year, I had found the community I was searching for. I cried a lot in the privacy of our apartment for months, hiding my pain from everyone, yet, not for my son's diagnosis, but more because of the unknown that lay ahead. Until this party I kept hearing all of the things Taylor wouldn't be able to do instead of what he could do. But these were all regular kids; they looked different than other children, but they seemed more loving and carefree than most typical children. It was a whole new world, and little by little, I was entering it.

I learned of the Early Start program in Southern California and called to arrange Taylor's first evaluation with a team of teachers and therapists who were a part of a local elementary school not far from where we lived. Pamela Ross, R.N., was our nurse and service coordinator. She came to our apartment on Boulder Avenue in January with a wonderfully kind woman named Prem Patel who would be Taylor's O.T. (Occupational Therapist). They did a full consultation and evaluation of Taylor and developed his first IFSP (Individualized Family Service Plan). The IFSP's are a love-hate in my world as they are a constant reminder of everything my child is working on to accomplish everyday life skills.

The IFSP forms would be used until Taylor reached the age of three, and then beyond age three they became IEP's (Individualized Education Plans). Both the IFSP's and the IEP's would be used for all of the years Taylor attended school, listing all of the goals and objectives that his team would be working on with him from self-help skills to building independence, to his every day academics. Reading the forms and understanding them can take years of trial and error because more often than not, the educators aren't helpful in guiding parents through each goal, objective and what they all meant at the end of the day. Still, they are crucial to the charting of expectations and goals for the development of each child, both at home, and in an educational system.

My most important concerns at the time in Taylor's IEP were being knowledgeable about what would help Taylor and for him to have as much of a normal life as possible. I thought these objectives were pretty simple, partly because I didn't know what to ask for, and partly because I had no idea what Taylor would and would not be able to do.

With the instruction of Prem Patel, we began simple massaging techniques to help build Taylor's low muscle tone, and I began the quest for toys that would stimulate his mind and grab his attention. They taught me a ton of fine motor skill exercises to begin building Taylor's cognitive behavior and abilities to use in everyday tasks, as well as the beginning stages of oral motor skills to strengthen his tongue muscles to not only retract voluntarily, but also give stability for future chewing and speaking. They guided me through his nutritional needs as well as the physical and mental transitions necessary in caring for him. At the same time they gave me courage through their knowledge and experience that Taylor would progress just as any other child, with a little more time and some extra help.

As much as I tried to adjust to our town in Southern California, I just couldn't. I was falling into an even deeper depression and missed the friends and familiarities of our suburban town in Northern California. After several months, Taylor and I made the leap and transferred back, reinstating all of his doctors and therapists. I loved the Bay Area and the access to Tahoe as well as the conglomeration of universities, research facilities and the lure of such a culturally diverse metropolitan city. I needed the familiar infrastructure of our local hospitals and trusted therapists that were so easily accessible. We needed to get him up to speed for his age and I felt in the long term, being back in our familiar surroundings and amongst friends would benefit both of us.

I was still traveling doing overnight flights for meetings to the East Coast for the small design project in Rhode Island, sometimes leaving from San Francisco to Newport in the morning, having my meeting at the client's home and flying back out that evening. My mother was a saint for these trips, flying from Southern California to San Francisco to watch Taylor and flying home the next day.

Many events between Taylor's birth until about the age of six months are still a blur. The few memories I do have involve attorney's fees I could barely pay and a crushing debt from moving and medical bills. Although I still have no idea other than a gift from God how it happened or how I got in touch with them, California Children's Services, came completely out of the blue and covered all of the costs from Taylor's birth. I had never transferred any legal authority over to my husband including my name and any bank or credit accounts because there was always so much chaos, it never felt safe to do so. So without my ability to contribute, CCS covered $86,000 for my emergency c-section as well as the eight days of Taylor's stay in the NICU. Every time I write a check to the state of California or to the I.R.S. for taxes I know why and am eternally grateful as a U.S. citizen for emergency programs like the ones that helped me. It can happen to any of us.

Financially, I took a hit for many years to come choosing to stay home with Taylor for the first eighteen months. I researched every available therapy, technique and skill known to help Taylor learn to walk, eat and excel wherever he could. In signing off from any child support, the only income I could bring in was from my small design project, as well as a little from the SSI Fund. I was constantly reminded by my family and friends to go back to his paternal father for child support, but my son's safety and well being as well as the psychological toll it would take on me having to re-live the darkness I had long ago left behind prevented me. So instead, we relied on help from family, friends and a few local groups when it came to groceries, clothing, etc.

I remember being so hungry—walking by restaurants and smelling the food, my stomach growling—and watching everyone eating. There were countless times of giving up my food in order to feed Taylor, but I didn't care because it was what you did as a mother. We tried one local food program where they asked what Taylor's diet was. I explained the only foods he would eat were pureed and only five different kinds, all a part of his oral aversions. They delivered an entire meal mashed up in a tall Styrofoam container for him, and wilted brown lettuce with something unidentifiable in a square Styrofoam container for me. I couldn't eat it nor could I imagine giving Taylor his.

So this was the welfare help politicians were referring to when running for re-election, I thought. Their views of supporting those in society unable to support themselves was so incredibly unrealistic and distorted. Inedible food that seemed to be leftovers from a restaurant dumpster were my former tax dollars hard at work, only this time I was on the receiving end, and it wasn't pretty. I was beginning to see the other side of life which millions of men, women and children were living every day of their lives.

We tried for another state program called WIC where they would furnish you as a new mother without sufficient income: diapers, portions of milk, bread, cheese and infant formula. I began to wonder how I was going to survive under the circumstances and how I was going to provide for my son, pay for a sitter and look for a job.

I had been a well-educated, accomplished, thirty-four year-old businesswoman just three years ago I with an average salary of $375,000 per year during the mid 90's. And now, I had nothing left in savings, nothing left on my credit cards and I was falling further and further behind in rent. All the while, I was also slowly losing my identity though all of these crises. I never pictured myself in this state of dependency and poverty. Nor did I look the part when walking into any state welfare office.

All I was seeing in the news day after day were the cuts to the very programs I was trying to support my son through. I imagined how many other children and families were going to be impacted. I'm not sure how legislators can stop funding programs for the underprivileged or say so many are "just living off of the system." Do the underprivileged not have equal value? Where has the compassion for our fellow neighbor gone? What was the true cost of the medications I couldn't afford for my son? And when was the last time they adjusted the poverty level requirements to balance the expenses of today's cost of living? The questions kept swirling in my mind. It made me realize how sheltered my life was before Taylor, and how lucky I was to have had the opportunities, in scholarships for college, family and friend's connections and my career. My whole life, I had worked as hard as I possibly could, paid enormous amounts in taxes, and done what I was told to do according to society's expectations. Now, it felt like I was on the other side of the fence in my very own country. I was just trying to understand and work through the red tape of life in supporting my son without a job, food and the possibility of becoming homeless because I was so far behind in rent.

At the end of the day all of my sacrifices both financially and socially were still worth it, and with each new day, I kept pushing forward against the odds because my son needed me to. I believed everything would eventually work out if I just kept focusing on the good and creating a positive and stable world for him against the odds. I'm not sure how he did it every day, but his smiles and laughter gave me a level of strength and courage I had never known I had, which in turn gave me a different level of tenacity in our survival. I could do anything if I just put my mind to it, and if I for a minute ever doubted myself, I remembered his sparkling blue eyes and his smile that seemed to shine to the moon and back.

I enrolled Taylor in The Early Start program through our local Regional Center for ages birth to three. This was the same program as Southern California, in which the many therapists either came to our home, or we went to their offices. From Speech, to Occupational Therapy to Physical Therapies, whatever it took, my mind was always open and so were my ears in providing resources to build Taylor's skills and independence. The Regional Center was an amazing resource and umbrella for funding all of Taylor's early intervention, and there is no way I could have done it without them. Again, this was another lifeline for knowledge and help and words cannot express how grateful I am to this very day for all that they did for Taylor during his most crucial developmental years. Every day we worked on his ability to walk, feed himself and talk so that as he became older we wouldn't need to rely so much on the system and the many therapists within it; instead he would use his learned skills, applying them both at home and within the community. I had learned to set small personal goals for both of us, taking it day by day, working on his present and future independence by finding his strengths and weaknesses and nourishing them both.

His oral aversions to food were becoming an extraordinary challenge when beginning to move him from breast milk to cereal from a spoon, to toddler bite size pieces of various foods. He would progress to pureed avocado and squash, and then divert back to cereal after any cold, flu or digestive illness. Five steps forward and four back was our progress on most given days, but I never stopped trying, because eventually I believed he could do it with my help. One of the most difficult times for any mother is when we don't think our children are getting enough nutrition, and I was no different in worrying. I read every book, sought every therapist known not only in our surrounding areas but throughout the country to figure out how to help him overcome his feeding challenges and food aversions. Mostly trying to work with his mouth through small chewy toys, and even a little Z-Vibe which was a toothbrush-like vibrator to stimulate and strengthen the low muscle tone within his mouth. Little by little, like a bird, he trusted me as he ate, although all on his time, certainly not mine. As we grew together during his different obstacles, I realized just how much patience and guidance he needed and how solid of a parent he needed me to be.

Before he turned a year old, we used as much food play as possible to build his awareness of textures. Even if he couldn't put it in his mouth, at least he could touch it, feel it and trust it. In therapy, we used the sand box, walking on grass, even a brushing technique to build his sensory awareness through his hands, feet, arms and legs. The technique was called the Wilbarger technique and used the same brush as the one we used in the NICU to wash our hands, with super soft bristles. With a downward motion on his arms, legs and back we gave gentle rhythmic strokes, avoiding the belly. It created sensory stimuli and he seemed to really like it. 1-2-3 strokes. Everything became 1-2-3 in most of the work with him because it created the known of a beginning expectation as well as an end for him.

In our first year together, we both accomplished so much, physically, mentally and spiritually, that I was becoming prouder and prouder of both of us as a team. At six months he was able to roll over. At nine months he was able to sit up and showed signs of wanting to crawl. We added a lot of ball therapy to his physical therapy sessions because the movement created a sense of fun while building his core strength. His muscle tone was very weak due to the hypotonia (low muscle tone) of Down syndrome, yet through repetition of certain core strengthening exercises, he slowly began to make huge leaps in progress. At fifteen months he was eagerly and quickly crawling all over the house and I have to say the fastest crawler I had ever seen! Once he began to realize he could get to where he was focused on going to, there was no stopping him.

It was so gratifying watching him try to accomplish even the simplest of tasks and watching him smile a mile long when he succeeded. His happiness was a ray of sunshine for everyone he came in contact with. I just wanted to help him more so he didn't feel he had to struggle to please me or anyone else, believing for the both of us that it all would flow naturally, eventually. Nothing was ever taken for granted and every accomplishment and success was appreciated and praised like there was no tomorrow.

The most difficult part still was not the doctor's visits, the therapies, his vulnerability to illness with a weak immune system, or the sleepless nights of worry over him. It was the stares by others that I saw, even though Taylor didn't notice or would comprehend at such a young age. The pain a parent holds when his or her child wasn't accepted or worse yet, made fun of, was a pain I never thought I would live through. While some comments were out of curiosity, most were just rude, cutting me to the core every time.

The worst was on a trip to my client's home in Rhode Island. I had taken the red eye to Newport for a meeting at her home, and was flying back out to San Francisco that night. We were standing in her kitchen reviewing my latest designs, when she blurted, "I am so sorry your son has Mongolism. Oh," she quickly retracted, "I'm sorry, they don't call them that anymore, do they?" My knees seemed to buckle and I lost my breath. I didn't know what to say. Especially because this project was our only source of real income; I bit my tongue and reminded myself money doesn't buy class and if anyone was that ignorant, words didn't need to be spoken to give credence to such a ridiculous and heartless statement.

Whether a child has cancer, a heart defect, or uses a wheelchair or communication device, whatever the cause, whatever the impairment, they are human beings first and foremost and should be treated equal, if not with a greater awareness and compassion because it takes that much more to do the things we take for granted.

The label was what I was finding was our biggest combatant. Living beyond the label was easy, but living within the label in the beginning was painful and difficult. Whenever I see parents with children who have special needs, my heart breaks knowing how hard so many of them work every day for their children, to give them the best that life has to offer with little personal respite. I wish people really knew more of their daily lives and struggles. Because in the end, a parent with a child who has special needs just wants love for his or her children and to fit in with his or her children as any other family: to be accepted without a label.

CHAPTER 4

Hope

When I was thirteen years old, I nannied for an amazing family in the Northeast at their country home during the summers. The wife, a beautiful model in New York City, and her husband, an incredibly intelligent investment banker, were just beginning their lives together. Their first born child who I had the honor of caring for, Megan, was the sweetest most angelic little girl with beautiful curly blonde locks. Two years later, her little brother Charlie came along. He, like his sister had a clump of curls at the base of his neck and the most irrepressible smile with an unbelievable amount of love and adoration for his mother. They were the beginning of my own hopes and desires to raise a family and have such beautifully perfect children. I loved them like my own and would do anything for them. They gave me a pseudo home without ever even knowing just how dysfunctional my own home life had been and the fear that I lived in daily between my father and brother. A long blonde haired country girl from the rolling lush green hills of the Northeast they thought, and for whatever reason, they gave me my first break in life and I'll never forget it. They gave me hope that someday my life would look like the same beautiful picture I had painted of their lives as a family filled with love, affection, kindness, and respect instead of the darkness of my own personal life with my family.

After twenty-eight years, they are still a very large part of my life. They invited Taylor and I for a long weekend just before Taylor's second birthday to their home in Florida. A dear friend of theirs, Ellie was a speech pathologist and had heard Taylor was having walking issues as well as feeding and speech problems.

His hypotonia was not an end all, rather he just needed a little more time and help to build his muscles and understand his movements and control thereof. So, Ellie arranged for Taylor to be seen by a team at the Dan Marino's Children's Hospital in Miami, which was basically a one stop shop for feeding, speech, occupational and physical therapy.

We arrived on an insanely hot tropical Thursday morning packed and ready for the day. For six hours Taylor was seen by the best team I had ever witnessed. Our feeding evaluation was twelve pages alone with answers and recommendations I still use. For him to understand the feeling of walking, they put Taylor into a small harness attached to a curved metal stand which sat on top of a slow moving treadmill. He was so cute in his surfer shorts, tee shirt, little leather Robbie shoes and white hair. The smile was as wide as the Florida sands—he was so proud of himself and the feeling of walking.

One of the best parts of the journey was my father's offering of financial help when I realized the best day of our life in building five different kinds of evaluations wasn't covered under our insurance. Even with a special rate, it was over a thousand dollars. Once again, the humiliation rose within me. One step forward and several back due to our lack of healthcare and steady income. It was clear I needed to get back to working full time and try to find a balance in all of the juggling. Within the next month or so, thanks to the trip to The Dan Marino facility and their guidelines, Taylor was now walking, showing independence, and mature enough health-wise to go into a day care program.

This was the real beginning of my anxieties. I had to leave him for at least six hours each day to complete strangers. I do realize most women had to do this just after their maternity leave was finished, and I give them the utmost respect. I wouldn't have been strong enough emotionally to let go at that time, especially with all of the therapies and medical issues we faced on a daily basis. Staying home with Taylor in our first two years together may not have been the best for us financially, but it made all the difference in the world in his progress and independence.

As I began to comb through a step-by-step plan, I realized even if I found a job, it would take some time to be able to build up enough money to support a babysitter or day care program, let alone a daycare program that would accept a child with special needs. Finally after weeks of research, I found a facility funded by the state. After several attempts and applications, I kept getting denied. When I finally pushed for answers at the main office and asked why we weren't eligible, they explained I was on a wait list and the criteria was based on a point system. Although income wise I was eligible, I wasn't a minority or recovering from an alcohol or drug addiction, so therefore, my points weren't qualifying me for Taylor's entry. Only after explaining that Taylor had special needs did they approve him for free day care so I could go back to working a full-time job. I could then eventually afford a private sitter who could give Taylor the extra attention he needed, as well as take him to all of his therapies, and doctor's visits.

However, after a bit of time in the program, another mother with a little girl with Down syndrome and I discovered no one had any experience with children with special needs. I was given daily sheets chronicling his feedings, diaper changes, etc. but not until I adamantly requested the details. When I asked what Taylor's activities were, they said brightly; "He is the perfect child! He will sit in a corner for hours and just look at books". Okay—let's get something straight, a child with Down syndrome or any child with special needs requires a completely different level of care. He needs more stimulation and more interaction not less. It was a free program, and my hands were clearly tied as no matter what I asked for, the bottom line was that no one had any experience with special needs and so it was easier to just ignore the children with special needs if they weren't aggressively acting out.

A small consolation was that his therapists were able to work with him in a back hallway of the day care once a week. His occupational therapist Allen was our most reliable and most comforting resource and Taylor absolutely adored him. Speech and feeding therapy however, I still had to work into my hectic work schedule and drive him to the therapist's office on the other side of town.

I had finally found a full time job and I hoped it would allow me to eventually pull Taylor out of the state-funded day care program and find a private facility or private sitter where he would receive the best of care. I remember as clear as if it were yesterday standing in front of the church where the day care was, negotiating my contract with an unknown Italian woman over my cell phone. She was the Vice President at the time of one of the most renowned wholesale design showrooms in the U.S. and it was an honor to even be on a list of possible candidates. I had found the small ad on Craigslist in which they were hiring an outside sales representative. I had no idea what that meant, but I knew the company, its reputation and knew more than anyone how to sell myself. I was maxed out on credit cards just trying to buy food, and the rent was two months behind. I was on the verge of losing everything; I needed this job for Taylor—no wasn't an option.

I had figured out where the showroom was in the Design District on the south side of San Francisco, and with the help of an old suit from my single and financially successful days, I pulled it out from under the dust and put it on. I found an old Hermes chocolate brown and black silk scarf, tying it Euro style around my neck with the tallest heels I could wear, for height always gave me an air of confidence. I needed to sell myself and my sense of style to the showroom manager, and at the end of the meeting, it must have worked. I was now having the conversation with the Italian woman from corporate headquarters over the phone, speaking so fast I didn't quite understand what she said, except sight unseen by her, I was hired. Salary, commission and health insurance!

Along with the waves of joy I now had to learn to balance working full-time with my constant priority, Taylor. My commute into the city was about forty-five minutes each way several times per week and, my territory as an outside sales person consisted of all Northern California from Carmel to Chico as well as Lake Tahoe and Nevada.

Traveling to Reno, Fresno, or any corporate meetings in Chicago or New York was an even greater challenge when my office required it. We often flew to my mother's in Southern California so she could watch him, toting all of the necessary essentials for his stay and my travels. While pushing Taylor in his stroller, I would carry the car seat, two suitcases, handbag, briefcase and case full of my fabrics to sell shuttling through the airport like a pack mule.

As time went on, the more I traveled without Taylor, flying became an even greater anxiety. Every takeoff and landing without Taylor I would pray to him "I will be home soon baby, I promise". The concerns of not having a solid back-up plan if something happened to me plagued my mind. I had never been a paranoid person, nor had I ever known what a panic attack was. Now I did. I didn't have life insurance, a savings account, a Will nor anyone to leave Taylor to as his legal guardian, and it was a nightmare of emotions every time I flew. I was growing accustomed to living pay check to pay check, and at least we had one, but the many anxieties of coordinating all of the travel, and everything I was trying to do became almost unbearably exhausting at times.

The constant worry of what happened to Taylor when I wasn't around him never subsided. When Taylor was at the state funded day care, we took many steps backwards in his development. To this day, I have terrible fears about Taylor's every day care, stemming from this almost two year experience at the day care program. I worry if he is getting the right care and is he safe? I worry he isn't getting enough attention and that his programs aren't directed or monitored by people that have experience, trained to handle children that are intellectually or developmentally challenged.

Our small town just outside of San Francisco was known to be in the top five for public schools in the entire state of California. Thankfully, Taylor was now old enough to enter pre-school. This should be an easy transition, right? Except for two things: we didn't have a pre-school in our wonderful little town, nor did I have a typically developing child that could go into a regular pre-school program.

So, we began the process of investigating our options. Taylor was still having a lot of problems transitioning, eating, still wasn't verbal, and was extremely sensitive to loud noises. Our Regional Center gave us the option of a small pre-school for children with various disabilities. It was about twenty miles northwest of us in the completely opposite direction of my work commute, however, like everything else, I would figure it out and adapt both of us to the situation. I agreed to take a tour and meet the teacher and team for Taylor's possible placement. I arrived at a quiet, long hallway with classrooms on either side. I remembered this same feeling as a child, with the smell of juice boxes, play dough and chalk. A typical school with schedules and artwork lining the walls, and yet, it wasn't your typical school. Its floors were lined with wheelchairs, walkers and devices for children to get from class to class. The tears welled in my eyes. How lucky were we that we didn't need them . . . . but I must be in the wrong place. This isn't my child. He doesn't belong here. Or, does he? Was he really in this category of disabilities? Was this the rest of my life with him? Doctors, therapists, hospitals and wheelchair lined halls in his school? In a split second I felt sorry for myself and for my life, but most of all for my son I treated like any other child. He had no label in my world. He was Taylor. Minute by minute, step by step I slowed my mind do be able to cope. *I have to make it to the classroom and meet his team, after all it was where everyone said that Taylor needed to be.* If I ever got scared in dealing with times like these, I learned to pretend I was going into a business meeting with the same air of confidence—like I knew what I was doing. It gave me courage to deal as a businesswoman, never allowing anyone to see me sweat.

No one seemed to have the answers and there didn't seem to be a lot of research-based information out there dealing with the various disabilities of our children. I had read and re-read every book I could find on feeding, speech, fine motor skills, gross motor skills, hypotonia, behavior, every medical journal, research, new trial for building cognitive behavior, advocacy, how to read an I.E.P, (Individualized Education Plan) and the occasional blog of a parent that was sharing their story so I didn't feel so alone. I tried to remember to re-group, especially when I had to hear another doctor tell me "It's behavioral" and "You need to start seeing a different team. This is their phone number, and oh by the way, it isn't covered under your insurance so you'll have to self pay." Or, "Oh yes, your son really needs speech therapy and perhaps feeding therapy as well, and oh, by the way, that isn't covered under your insurance either." I reminded myself there would be easier times ahead as Taylor became more independent and better educated. I'd be lying though if I didn't admit how much I prayed for a place where we would have reliable help, and where I personally wouldn't be alone forever in this amazing journey, instead sharing it with someone special. Day by day I kept imagining a life beyond the walls I was living behind. Someday I would find a place where I wouldn't have to fight for help for my son at every turn, for my son to be accepted at school and throughout his community without hesitation. A place where we could just be, without everyone staring because we were a little different.

As I reflect back, Taylor has saved my life in many ways beyond the obvious, and I see the world completely differently now. Trying to find answers when I think all I really need to do is curl up with Taylor and read a good Dr. Suess book together or go to the park and just play. Maybe sometimes, it's not so important that I have all of the answers but rather start living and actually enjoying the life that we do have and all of the things we can do. My circle of friends and family is extremely tight and I only surround myself with the positives in life. It became the only way I could gather my strength for us on a daily basis. Through his eyes, it's all about play, having fun, creating and enjoying the simplest of things in life: throwing rocks in the water or going for a long walk in the woods. He is his best in naturally quiet environments and thrives in the outdoors. He adores swimming, horseback riding and riding his bicycle just like any child. Funny, it's no different than what I like to do, however I find myself getting too caught up in the minutiae of the everyday, exhausted and worrying about everything for him. I look forward to living and seeing more of life through his eyes and really getting to know everything about him. He's quite fascinating to watch and get to know as a person, and I grow more and more intrigued by the ways in which he communicates as a non-verbal child. Getting to know more about his beautiful idiosyncrasies, mannerisms and gestures will only bring us closer as well as help me to provide him with the ability to communicate effectively with his peers. It's a lifelong experience that I look forward to, developing by his side so he never thinks he's different, but instead is respected and accepted amongst his peers.

I look back now in writing this and want to honor every parent that has lived this day: the day you realize the reality of your life in the present moment and just how difficult these times were. My highest respect and love for every parent and child that is bound to the adversities they didn't ask for, and may the adversities not define us, but challenge us to be who we always wanted to be in the eyes of our children and ourselves. The knowledge lies within each moment, in how to deal with the bad and embrace the good to make a better tomorrow for those who face the same.

CHAPTER 5

Tenacious

For the first few weeks, I drove Taylor to school every day and walked him into the classroom in hopes of transitioning him without a crying episode. I found the most important thing for him was structure, sticking to the routine with little deviation. It was always heart wrenching dropping him off as I rushed to work, hearing him cry so hard it was as if he thought I might never return. All the professionals I knew told me his new little preschool was the best place I could put Taylor for his capabilities. He wasn't showing any signs of verbalizing to communicate, didn't know or understand sign language, nor did he have any interest in learning signing just yet. He wasn't ready to be potty trained, and his lack of fine motor and gross motor skills put him at a six month to one-year-old level according to their evaluations. He was now four years old. So, as the professionals said, this school housing just children with disabilities is the best place possible for him to learn and thrive both academically and in building his future life skills.

I found the most difficult part in transitioning him to this special school, was convincing me that this was the best placement for his education. After two weeks, he seemed to have formulated a routine within the classroom. He appeared to be content in the class until 12:45 at which point the teacher would place him and another student into a little red Radio Flyer wagon and roll them over to a day care until I could pick him up at 5:30. He seemed to acclimate to his new routine and environment much faster than any of us could have imagined. I was the one that had to live with all of the reports, evaluations and recommendations of those that I knew in my small circle of professionals who all said my son needed a school for children with varying levels of severe to not so severe learning disabilities, rather than a regular school with typically developing children. I was living with my new reality, not the protected and somewhat sheltered life I chose to live within before all of this. Or was it? I treated him like any other typically developing child, however, here he was put into a box where everyone thought children that had moderate to severe disabilities needed to be in an institutionally-based style of learning. I had no instruction book, so I followed the recommendations.

His arrival was at 8:45 every day when he was eventually expected to unpack his back pack, hang up his jacket, and then have both free choice and some directed play. 9:45 was clean up and the ability to follow directions related to the daily routine. 9:55 morning circle of songs, greetings and welcome activities. 10:05 learning activity centers which consisted of ten minute activities with children all rotating in groups. One would be based on language expansion and the second on fine motor skills. 10:35-11:00 Recess. 11:35-11:55 Bathroom and free play activities. Tuesdays and Wednesdays 11:45-12:30 they had sensory motor group with the Occupational Therapists. This was basically miscellaneous gross motor skills emphasizing balance, perceptual motor coordination, and developmental movement skills as well as selected fine motor table activities. 12-12:30 Table activities and various structured group activities. This consisted of various art projects, reinforcing monthly colors or shapes, the current vocabulary unit, or just fun time. The more structured group activities were story times, music and fine and or gross motor activities. 12:30-12:45 Closing circle where they sung the good-bye song and each child would be excused.

It all sounded so perfect, regimented with enough play and instruction involved; therefore it must be the right place for him. On average there were twelve to fourteen children with Down syndrome, and moderate levels of other cognitive developmental challenges. There was one main teacher with two aides. For the first few months I seemed to be in a fog just trying to coordinate everything, be on time, rush to the city, out of the city, and pack in all of my road travel and client calls before the end of the day. My car flew along the highway more often than not, wheels barely hitting the pavement at the end of the long day because, inevitably, I was late from a client or just merging through heavy Bay Area traffic. I pushed my station wagon like it was a high performance car, praying to not get speeding tickets or worse, get in an accident.

I just wanted Taylor to be happy in his new school and for both of us to acclimate to this new world of a child that may or may not produce and articulate his speech, eat what most children eat, as well as simple tasks like transitioning from one place to another. I would be happy if he would at least try ice cream, whip cream, anything. But, I always had to remind myself, *it's not about me dragging him into my world with expectations of all of the things that come with it; perhaps the expectations are just too much for him at the time.*

I found myself becoming more of a recluse amongst my own friends as time went on. Our worlds didn't seem to relate much to each other any more. Explaining our every day or even a simple conversation with anyone was more of a work out because I had to explain everything as an outsider in so they could understand, rather than openly talk about it. The last thing I wanted was for anyone to say the words, "I'm sorry" or to have any kind of pity for having a child that wasn't "perfect" or that was "different". Birthday parties were extremely difficult because he wasn't able to filter the noise, and we couldn't do play dates because he didn't have the capacity to play and interact with typical peers at his current developmental level. All he knew were the wide range of children with various disabilities and behavioral issues from his preschool, rather than the expected behavior to which he would have seen if he were around typically developing peers.

After a few months, it became apparent there were some pretty serious issues within his classroom, and Taylor was beginning to show some behavioral problems at home as well as within the school. The powers that be were even questioning if he needed to be placed into a more severe range of the children with Autism classroom. As time went on, he wasn't transitioning as easily as we had initially thought and the teacher and aides were having to physically move him from place to place because he was refusing to move. One child consistently hit him and seemed to be bullying him, often coming home with bite marks and scratches. He would choose a toy and find the quietest, most hidden corner of the classroom as a safety net. The teachers ignored him, not even attempting to pull him back into the classroom to interact with them or his peers because he was being, "a good little independent boy". What it really meant was that he was isolating himself from the bullying, yelling and crying of the other children, and completely regressing socially and academically by hiding in the corners of the classroom. At home, he was beginning to bite me and act out in ways I had never seen before. He is the most non-aggressive child, always choosing to walk away from a situation versus confront or hit, push or bully back.

His clothing and face were smeared with the occasional phlegm of a runny nose and his diaper was consistently wet whenever I or his occasional babysitter Anjelina made an early and unannounced pick-up. The teachers faces by the end of their day looked like they had lived through a battle, and in a way, they did with so many children and so little of an infrastructure to help them. They were so overwhelmed and it was becoming a huge safety issue for each and every child as well as the teachers. There was near chaos every day with the lack of help for so many developmentally-challenged children, all bottled up in one small classroom. As the year went on, the levels of behavioral issues were heightened and getting much worse and more aggressive. They were all modeling after one another's bad behaviors, frustrated from the lack of prompting from one task or transition to another. Most lacked verbalization so there was no efficient way to communicate other than aggressive and sometimes hurtful actions to gain attention.

I inquired about Taylor's daily behaviors and the teacher and aides said he mostly played by himself in a quiet corner although he was well aware of his peers and his teachers and loved to watch them play from a distance. When the class transitioned outside to play, the teacher reported that they had to physically and verbally guide him outside instead of him initiating any independence. Throughout the day he sought out different ways to sooth himself, pressing his body up against a soft couch then repetitively climbing onto the couch, and sliding off of it. He frequently spun in a circle with his eyes closed with his hands propped in front of him as he spun as if he were peering through his fingers to see the patterns within. He sought out vestibular input as much as possible, because it was how he self-soothed and self-regulated within the chaos of the classroom that surrounded him.

I really believe this is why Taylor progressed so little during this time period. He was moved from station to station without prompting or with little to no one-on-one attention because they were so overwhelmed by the lesser functioning children. If they had more teachers and or an additional aides, the dynamics of each child would have completely changed, and I bet each child would have been more well-behaved and receptive to learning. The teacher and aides were all being reactive to the entire environment rather than proactive because they didn't have the necessary tools to succeed.

I had called meetings with the principal of the school, and requested numerous times another aide for the classroom. The staff couldn't handle the child to teacher ratio. Over and over I was bullied into accepting the excuse of extreme budget issues, and that the ratio was acceptable within the policies and guidelines of the school. I knew it wasn't right. None of it was. But what could I do? What, if any, choices did I have? This was completely unchartered territory for me and I didn't know how to push, when to push or felt comfortable enough to know I could push for more for my son, let alone the entire classroom

By February nothing had changed, except that I was having so many odd behaviors coming out of Taylor I sought the guidance of a behaviorist at home, to no avail. Unless someone went to the classroom and observed, there was no real logical approach to understanding where the behavior was coming from. Finally, with the addition of yet another student mid-February, I had had enough. They weren't adding another teacher or aide, and it was not acceptable to me any longer. I had a final meeting with the principal, where he gave me my options. I could call for a Mediation and Alternative Dispute Resolution in which I could ask the district to resolve the situation in mediation and it wouldn't delay my right to a due process hearing. Then, if mediation didn't result in hiring an additional aide for the classroom, we would have to have a due process hearing under the following categories for cause: the identification of my child for special education eligibility, the assessment of my child, the educational placement of my child, and, the provision of a free appropriate public education (FAPE) for my child. So, I cut to the chase after so much bureaucracy and frustration and requested a hearing. I thought the principal's eyes would burn a hole in me and his attitude of discontent was quite clear. How dare I challenge his direction and decisions within the school? But I didn't care what he thought. My son was in a negative situation and as a hard working, tax paying citizen of the United States, darn if I was going to sit back and just take it. I worked too hard to get to this point. My son has every right as a citizen of this country to be treated with dignity and respect.

And so, after weeks of back and forth conversations and letter writing to the various school heads, a meeting was scheduled to sit down and discuss the problem. As the school was in a different district, we called upon a representative from my small town for her presence and input. If another aide was going to be implemented into Taylor's classroom, then my district would have to pay for it according to this school. It was becoming clear that at the end of the day it was all about money, and always would be within the educational system. I had no idea what I was doing, I just knew the children in the classroom and my son were not being properly cared for and the teacher and aides needed help. So, I put my suit on and grabbed the two-inch file of documentation and headed into the district Educational Department offices.

The Director of Special Education for the county, the principal, recorder, the representative from my school district and I all sat around a large table with all of our files. The conversation went in circles for what seemed like forever to establish the ratio of teachers and aides to students. Not what was appropriate for the children and staff, but the numbers according to the county. What they weren't addressing was the success rate of each child's learning outcomes or if the system was working for each individual child as a whole, let alone the various safety issues. The classroom was chaotic to say the least and the educational setup was detrimental to any possible success for each individual child. Children hitting each other, not being kept clean, and being restrained were not acceptable within any classroom. And certainly not my son's.

Stephanie Simms was the Special Education Director sent on the behalf of my district school. I had never met this woman before, and I figured she would be someone else I would have to fight, but looking back, she was our first real angel. She very diplomatically addressed all of the concerns and bullet pointed how she saw a sufficient outcome in working with their school. She insisted another aide be placed into the classroom. Finally I thought, someone was on the same page as me, caring and hearing my voice. Advocacy for the first time in my life was a new word with a real definition. Someone was hearing my cries in the middle of the night, and my plea for a break.

The meeting was adjourned with the resolution that an additional aide would be placed in the classroom. We won! For all of those students whose parents couldn't find their own voices or just simply didn't know how or if they could ask, as well as their sons and daughters within Taylor's class. The district had to now fight as to who was going to pay for the aide. But, my part was done, and I had found a new friend for Taylor and me, someone who would understand and protect us in a sense. So crazy we had to fight for the obvious in a public school, and I wished so badly we could move Taylor somewhere that included him as in a regular classroom.

I still couldn't fully accept what all of the professionals were telling me. My son was not limited in his learning. He certainly had different needs with respect to how he was taught and how he learned, but my gut and observations for four years told me he had way more potential than anyone was giving him credit for. He just needed more support academically and socially. The increase of an aide to his classroom was a band aide. It wouldn't change the policies of the school, the district or how the daily curriculum adjusted to the needs of each child. On an everyday basis, he wasn't being challenged academically in the classroom and he wasn't being given the necessary tools to accommodate for his disability, so there was no way he could succeed under their platform. It made me start looking at the capabilities of all of the other children in his classroom rather than looking at their inabilities.

People were so quick to move my son into a box and stereotype, which only made me more curious as to just how many other students in the school were being stifled and not given the proper resources to see their true potentials. They would never know their true potentials, interests, or be able to thrive as most children hope to within the general education system without proper assessments, interventions and accommodations. Regardless of my son's diagnosis and all of the other children within his classroom, I truly believed the child should come first and the label or disability second.

Meanwhile, I was still dealing with the financial hardships. I had diligently investigated every possible resource for us financially. I was making too much money to continue receiving SSI, but I did qualify Taylor to receive Medical/Medicaid for life due to his permanent disability. There was talk of putting him on a feeding tube because he wouldn't eat anything beyond oatmeal for breakfast, a yogurt snack, a Pediasure shake and spaghetti for lunch and dinner. He was only in the 25th percentile for height and weight and marked as "failure to thrive" both nutritionally and due to his hearing loss in both ears. Thankfully, California Children's Services aided us again when the time came for him to go under anesthesia as an outpatient and have tubes put in both ears. I was working as hard as I possibly could, and we were barely getting by. I didn't have a home to re-mortgage and there was no family help, so I kept my chin as high as I could for the day this would all just be a bad memory and not our future reality.

We were maintaining though. I didn't go out on dates, or to the movies or even the occasional dinner out. Every day and night was spent caring for Taylor and trying to figure out how to get out of our hole. Work was picking up and my sales were rapidly increasing, but it wasn't enough. I began selling everything I could to pay off our debts from the first two years of staying home to care for Taylor and the attorney bills. From my kayak to road bike to some of my more expensive suits I had acquired in my career days before Taylor, and even my wedding ring.

From the time Taylor was six months old, my neighbor and now best friend Gavin had been bringing us groceries from our local Trader Joes when he knew I couldn't afford them. I believe he had heard a bit of my story, yet never asked and never questioned anything. He also never asked for anything in return, just to be a friend and was always eager to take a simple walk with Taylor and me through our neighborhood.

One of Taylor's greatest gifts is being able to connect with people on a higher level of spiritual thought rather than what I call the mundane-ness of our everyday life. Taylor's world is only of love, peace, laughter and the uncanny ability to always give you a hug when you or someone else needs it the most.

Our Regional Center service coordinator met with us every quarter to review Taylor's file. Through the coordinator, we were given Respite Care hours so I could have a much needed break, even something as simple as going to the grocery store or getting a hair cut was impossible without someone to watch Taylor. If

I wasn't working, Taylor was with me 24/7. So, we started at about fifty hours per month in which they would pay $10.39 per hour. After the hours had accumulated and I had paid the sitter, I would be reimbursed by a check for those hours on the 11th of the following month. It was a huge, huge help, but having to front the money until the middle of the next month was nearly impossible. We just didn't have the reserves, so I tended not to use it. I was given a tip by a dear friend for another program called In Home Support Services which is for the elderly and for those with disabilities. Although we were in a grey area of eligibility because of Taylor's age, after a careful review we met the criteria. Taylor wasn't able to feed himself by age four and a half, wipe his mouth, use the potty, or do any of the most common minimal self-care of children his age. And this was just a small portion of the list. A feeding tube would require twenty-four hour care.

Our other challenge and one of the most difficult was trying to find an inexpensive place to live within our suburban town outside of San Francisco. The prices weren't as much as the city, but close to it. Then, after more extensive research, I found a below market rate program and figured I was willing to try for anything if it bettered our lives and helped me to eventually access a debt-free life. The program offered housing units available for first time home buyers in the state of California who also met certain income criteria at below market rates. On July 7, 2007 I received a phone call that I had won the lottery and was one of ten people eligible for a small unit with two bedrooms. 756 square feet on the second floor including a small deck, and ironically, it was in the same neighborhood I had been living in. Okay—scream, scream, laugh, laugh. Unbelievable! As usual, I had no idea how I was going to pull it off, but I believed in myself and pushing to better Taylor's life and wouldn't take no for an answer. We had no money in savings and my credit rating was just fair. With the extraordinary help of my best friends Joe and Carmen, as well as some fancy paperwork from my mom, we qualified. It took about three months, and I think the mortgage broker was ready to kill me for my tenacity by the end, but Taylor

59

and I had a home of our own that we owned, and the mortgage payment was half of what people charged for rent. I realized I really could do anything with Taylor if I just put my mind to it, with a lot of hard work, determination and guts.

As for Taylor, his classroom received the aide within two weeks of our hearing, however, Stephanie Simms the Special Education Director was recommending an alternative. She had proven I could trust her with my son's care and her educational experience as well as kindness and the respect towards me as a parent allowed a dialogue no one in the educational system had offered before. What she suggested was my dream all along, and yet I was terrified the day she actually said the words: "How about putting Taylor into a regular kindergarten classroom?" she asked. My jaw dropped and I went into a cold sweat. Another change. Another transition for him, and in a regular classroom where he would be amongst regular children. They would provide an aide to help throughout his day and shadow him from 8 AM to 12:25; he would be amongst his typically developing peers learning beside them, playing with them and attending a regular school with most of the same regular school routines. It was the craziest thing I thought I would ever hear, yet in my heart, I knew this was right for Taylor.

I met Stephanie one morning and stood with her in the back of the classroom to observe another boy with Down syndrome sitting amongst his peers on the carpet participating and fully interacting with everyone in every capacity. He was happy, well-adjusted and as much a part of the classroom as any other child, and most importantly he was truly a child first. Not a boy with Down syndrome but a boy who happened to have Down syndrome. My vocabulary, knowledge and understanding of all people with disabilities was becoming more clear as well as respectful. He had a name, not a label within his classroom. His aide was off to the side, and would only intervene when he needed something a fellow peer couldn't help him with.

The thoughts of relief were overwhelming and I felt that I finally had hope again, and we now had a school and community that were willing to give my son a normal life. The emotions kept swirling through my mind as well as all of the natural fears any parent has when making a change for their child in a school environment. Could Taylor really do this with the proper team support and aide, and would he be capable of sitting comfortably in this type of environment? How would it benefit the other children in the classroom? As I glanced over at Stephanie, feeling her eyes on mine, I could tell this wasn't the first time she had seen the same look in other parent's eyes when suggesting their child with special needs be included in a general education classroom. I am sure in her thirty years of teaching, being a principal and now a Director, none of this was a new experience for her, and it bolstered my confidence in her. She knew what my son was capable of, and most of all she believed in his potential. She gave a reassuring nod and a strong arm around my shoulders. I let go. For once I let go of trying to control everything and I somehow had faith in this woman and I had an even deeper faith in my son. I had to let him go, and learn to intervene only when it was appropriate. A fine line for any parent. When do I get involved? Will I even be heard when I did speak up or would it always be a battle? And when would be the day come when I could just have faith in my son's education and the professionals within?

One thing I did know, my son deserved a chance. So, we began the process in March of 2008 by meeting with the superintendent of our local district and the principal of the school. I think we were all just listening and holding our breath at the same time. They were deeply committed to fully including children with disabilities into their school, and were willing under these most unusual circumstances, to include my son. It all begins at the top. It needed to begin with the superintendent who had over twenty years of experience in special education. She was a career educator and a mother. She got it. And the principal was one of the loveliest, soft spoken and bright women I had met within the system. They just wanted him in their classroom and to be a part of their school.

CHAPTER 6

Acceptance

On April 23, 2009 Taylor was registered at our local elementary school as a kindergartner. We all took a giant leap of faith and entered him five months before his sixth birthday. We still didn't have a pre-school program for the children in our district so enrolling Taylor early into kindergarten was our only choice.

Even though Taylor was very young for this particular classroom developmentally, he seemed to embrace it on many different levels. He was still completely non-verbal and required transition objects or photos to move from one place to the other within the classroom or around the school grounds, but he clearly felt included and seemed to transform into a different child within days of his start. The aide and teacher helped him with transitions by cuing him using pictures of where he was to go throughout the school environment. From the library to the playground, or to the computer lab, the pictures were used as prompts so he was aware of not only what was expected, but also that he had some personal and independent choices he could make at different times during his day. The pictures gave him somewhat of a voice without actually having one and helped him transition with more ease.

He had regressed terribly at the preschool, and had almost no peer interaction skills nor desires to interact. Putting him into a typical general education classroom even with an aide, was a gutsy risk for all of us and is not an ideal situation for every child, but for him it worked right from the start. Taylor's abilities rather than inabilities were becoming clear to me. None of us really knew just how much cognitive potential Taylor had until we tested, assessed, and observed him within his natural environments. Regardless of how big or how small the accomplishments were, I would never have known Taylor's true potentials and abilities until I gave him the tools, created a stable and safe environment, and allowed him his independence and freedom to be amongst his typical peers. Once I let go as a mother, and he was included in his general education classroom, he began to shine within his school and community because he was now modeling how the majority of society acted and conducted themselves in everyday life.

By day four, Taylor was almost completely transitioned and loving his classroom. His teacher had the patience of a saint. She had two boys with various levels of regressed cognition and twenty-two other students to contend with. However, she not only embraced it, but embraced Taylor for the brave little boy that he was at a very young age for her classroom. If Taylor cried when I dropped him off, by 10:30 a.m. that same morning, she was sending me photos via e-mail of Taylor playing or doing an activity with a peer. The tears welled in my eyes every time I got a new ping on my Blackberry. Each photo depicted him enjoying his new environment, and for a parent like me, it really was extraordinary especially after having lived through all of the horrors of the state-funded day care program, and then the "Institutionally based" preschool.

The understanding of what inclusion really meant was the most important part of the entire process in this new school in comparison to the last school's philosophy. The previous school believed their education of students was based on an early intervention program rather than a regular curriculum based general education school. In other words, the most fundamental years of a child's development were between ages birth and three. Hence, the Early Start Program we were a part of. Then, instead of introducing the child who has special needs to a regular pre-school environment around peers they could model verbally, socially, and cognitively, they isolated my son into a self-contained environment.

In many ways I felt I was dealing with the exact same issue of the 1960's: segregation. However, unlike the struggle championed by Martin Luther King Jr., the battle for children and people with disabilities was complicated by the fact that so many, like my son, did not have the power of their own voice, because they were non-verbal, perhaps without hearing, visually impaired, or simply too young to communicate properly in a socially segregated world. Children with disabilities went from being automatically sent to an institution after birth thirty years ago to today when families like mine were finally speaking up and bringing their children into their hearts, homes, and communities.

The more I researched and the more I spoke to various families with children with disabilities, the more I found much of the misconceptions of children's inabilities stemmed from their original doctor at birth and the medical field. I was finding there simply wasn't enough empirical evidence to provide better information to the doctors or parents about the child's abilities when they were given their label at birth. Countless doctors within the medical community after diagnosing a child with a disability led my friends down a really negative path often labeling them as "mentally retarded" and explaining all of the possibilities of complications both mentally and physically. And, more often than not, the doctors implied and even suggested aborting the child when the new pregnancy test results came back positive for Down syndrome. I often wondered how much differently my son would have been treated if he perhaps had cancer instead of an intellectual disability. Would society treat him differently and perhaps with more acceptance?

In my countless weeks, months and now years of research I came across two incredibly provocative YouTube videos that became the catalyst for my personal understanding and future advocacy of civil rights for those with intellectual disabilities. They showed The Willowbrook school in 1965. Both videos show not only the problems people with intellectual disabilities, past and present, endure in the United States, but also throughout the world.

We are one of the wealthiest and most socially developed countries in the world, and yet we have only started to view human rights for those with disabilities thanks to former President John F. Kennedy in 1965. He visited The Willowbrook State School in New York. The school was a state-supported institution for children with mental retardation located in the Willowbrook neighborhood of Staten Island in New York City from the 1930s until 1987. It was designed for 4,000, but by 1965 it had a population of 6,000. At the time it was the biggest state-run institution for the mentally handicapped in the United States; mostly children.

The videos for me, supported my fear and realization that it was a cultivation of years of segregation, dating back to the first asylum in 787 A.D. It wasn't until Queen Elizabeth's 1533-1603 monarchy during the Renaissance Era when she proclaimed it was the government's responsibility to take care of the mentally disabled. For hundreds of years, people with intellectual disabilities had been put into institutions and shunned from society. The ostracized children within the institutions when starved from stimulation would often hurt themselves to feel something, anything, when all they really wanted, like all of us as infants wanted, was love. The lack of attention and services for the intellectually disabled often times lead to a lifelong dependency on an already exhausted system rather than creating an infrastructure of support from the beginning to create independence and build their future life skills. So many of the families I had spoken with were caught in a spider web of educational bureaucracy, with a huge lack of quality trained teachers and general help for their children on a daily basis. I was searching for the answers to create a new paradigm of thought for people that did have intellectual or physical differences within society and to create a better understanding and therefore acceptance of them. Maybe not everyone would embrace my new paradigm, but perhaps my son could actually be the inspiration to show what could be . . .

I think back to the times when I sat across from a crying and distressed parent because they were in the midst of fighting with their local school to try to get a regular inclusive education for their child with a disability. So many of them were being intimidated by a teacher or like my case, the principal, into believing their child should be in a special classroom with other children with special needs rather than the general education classroom.

As I thought back over the years of more misconceptions of children with disabilities, another image popped into my mind. I had been traveling in some quite extensive social circles of "blue bloods" as well as extremely successful and privileged families for business and pleasure. I remember several of them joking about marrying the right person to have their perfect children and lineage. By marrying outside of their society or elite social circles, they became a target of social ostracism and eventually blacklisted. Not just for financial reasons, but also for the misconceptions and fears of creating a child that would not meet their social, physical, or intellectual standards.

No one in my entire family history has ever had an intellectual disability, and until there is more research as to the causes of children being born with Down syndrome, I hope others will respect and invest in that same research to prevent more misconceptions which only stigmatize. In my quest for a line of defense against the misconceptions, I had our DNA researched at Stanford University in California to better understand the reason, the cause. In reviewing the test results, they handed me an 8.5x11 white sheet of paper with little squiggles depicting our DNA and where the chromosomes had spilt which resulted in the label. It had nothing to do with lineage, or alcohol or marrying someone within my small town. It was a random split of a gene and I have to say I am actually really grateful for the split, because my son has made me personally the best person I could ever hope to be and I wouldn't change a minute of his life or mine because of it. He has taught me compassion, love, patience, and the ability to treat others the way I always wanted to be treated, all because of a tiny cell splitting. So instead of concentrating on what could have been, I focus on what is, who he is and embrace it with a different perspective and appreciation.

By Including Taylor in a main stream school, and through the support of a proper team of therapists and teachers, as well as an aide, he soared. He was now peer-modeled and peer-supported in his regular kindergarten classroom. If he needed a break with a task or center in the beginning days of kindergarten and his new environment, he was allowed to go outside walking hand in hand with a peer. Or, with any of his therapies, such as speech for example, he would walk with his peer and that peer would participate with him. So not only was Taylor getting the modeling thru the peer, the peer was also getting a one on one session with the speech therapist with Taylor, working on his or her own developing skills. Instead of him being singled out and "pulled" out of the classroom as a child with a disability, he had a buddy system that allowed both of them to access a different dimension of their education.

On an everyday basis, Taylor was as much a part of the classroom as any other child. As time progressed, the aide was able to back off and just shadow Taylor within the classroom, and the teacher took the lead with instructing the entire classroom including Taylor without a lot of extra effort because she adapted the classroom for all of the children. The aide assisted when his peers weren't capable, like opening one of his snack containers, or zipping a zipper, etc. as well as assisted the entire classroom as a whole, not just Taylor.

One of the greatest joys was seeing the children throughout the classroom become so much more enriched by the entire process of helping one another *because* of Taylor instead of *for* Taylor. The teacher had created an entire framework of positive behavior and peer-modeling so they helped one another throughout their day. In such an extremely diverse world, the teacher had taught each and every child in this wonderful little kindergarten classroom social-emotional integration skills and positive behaviors that they will use throughout their entire lives. Everyone in the entire classroom benefited that year on so many different levels because of an incredible teacher named Ms. Cadence. They learned compassion, integration, acceptance, and a better understanding of themselves with no bullying or teasing. It was our first introduction to true inclusion which wasn't a place, but a set of values and respect for one another.

CHAPTER 7

Balance

As Taylor was adjusting to his new world, I was trying my best to adjust to mine. Shortly after we won the Below Market Rate Lottery for our little condominium, I was promoted from outside sales person for our company, to Managing the showroom at the southern end of San Francisco. The promotion was an honor as I was only with them a short eight months before I was offered the position. The hours were more fixed from 8:45 to about 5:50 which was much easier than juggling all of the overnight outside sales trips, and long hours of my previous position as a sales girl. Best of all, the salary and commission structure was better for helping Taylor and me start the process of getting back on our feet financially. It came with a lot more pressure and responsibility, but at this point, I really felt after everything we had been through I could do anything and was afraid of nothing, except not being able to put food on the table and pay the mortgage.

The idea and possibility of the promotion all began at a national sales meeting at the corporate headquarters in Bethpage, New York. It would mean another juggle and expense of my mother flying to San Francisco and relieving me for a few days so I could fly to New York, but I knew it was worth the chance to invest the time and money in the trip. In complete confidentiality, I had requested to interview while I was there with the wonderful Italian woman that hired me over the phone for the original outside salesperson position. She agreed to the interview after many hours and weeks of talking about the position and mentoring me to see if I could handle the job. The numbers at the time were about $475,000 in revenue per month that I would be responsible for, plus the management of all eleven employees. The showroom wasn't doing well with the present manager, and they needed someone to completely re-vamp and possibly change all or part of the staff. I was entering the corporate world without ever having time to realize it; which was probably a good thing in retrospect. Had I realized how stressful it would all be, I probably would have thought harder in accepting it!

We arranged to meet after the corporate headquarters' meetings at Anthony Bourdain's bistro on Park Avenue on the upper Eastside of New York. I had stayed with my best friend in my childhood town the night before, and taken the bus in to meet her. I was on a shoestring budget, and needed to save every dime without it showing and the bus was the cheapest transportation to get to her for the meeting. I never went to sleep the night before, worrying about how badly I really needed this promotion. The money was of paramount importance, but also the boost to my self-worth.

Gabriella was the most beautiful, petite Italian woman I had ever met, and we sat for over two hours just talking. She chain smoked cigarettes as we drank our cappuccinos as if we were sitting in a piazza at a trattoria somewhere in Italy. It was a world away from my life back home feeling free of responsibilities or the worries of California even if for a couple of hours. In typical Italian fashion it was all about talking and getting to know one another beyond business and not until the last half hour of our meeting did we discuss the position. She was an inspiration as a businesswoman and perhaps one of the greatest mentors I had ever known. I worked for weeks trying to get to this point, and even after all of the caffeine, all of the talking, at the end, I still didn't know if I had gotten the job or not. I knew I was their best candidate with my years of experience in the design industry as well as a determination to succeed, but I also knew corporate was a completely different ball game and it could be smoke and mirrors at times with lots of promises and little delivery. She kindly explained that she had many people to report back to before I was given the go ahead and that she would be in touch soon.

I flew back to California that evening on pins and needles, still keeping everything including the meeting itself confidential from everyone back at the design showroom until I had been offered the job. Then, even if I did get the job, we had to wait for the corporate office to announce it to all of the showrooms throughout the country before I said anything to anyone. Every day that went by on my existing salary was agony as we lived paycheck to paycheck and I couldn't wait to start making more of a dent in the debt from the divorce attorney, medical bills, and life in California.

After three long weeks, they made me an offer, I accepted and it was formally announced. I was the new showroom manager to one of the most prestigious wholesale interior design companies in the country with a reasonable amount of an increase in salary so I could hire my existing babysitter on an almost full time basis. This was an accomplishment for both Taylor and me to work towards a better life for both of us with more money, and therefore more access to all of the therapies and services I couldn't presently afford for him.

However, as I was soon to discover, this is where things became even more complex. I was making more money, but the babysitter needed to work longer hours, eating into the extra money I was making. I couldn't afford just pulling two deductions, so I claimed five which began my tax implications of which I am still paying eight years later. I quite simply had no idea. The more money I made, the more I was taxed, and the more I was taxed, the farther into debt I was becoming. Not only was I now paying the sitter more, I was no longer being reimbursed for mileage to travel; so the almost $3.00 per gallon for roughly 58 miles per day across the bridge then across town was all mine. $6.00 to get over the bridge, plus $10.00 per day in parking. Daily it was about $22.00 per day just in commuting. However, in so many ways, it was much easier not only going to work in a nine to five job, but also having the support of a babysitter. Someone else to help so all of the responsibility in caring for Taylor didn't solely fall on me.

Our life was finally starting to normalize as much as expected. I dropped Taylor off at school every day at 8:00 am and rushed off to work in the city. He remained there until 12:25 pm when the sitter would pick him up, and take him to her home for lunch, nap and playtime. She has a wonderful little boy Brice who absolutely adored Taylor. She lived in the same home with her parents, son and husband so it gave Taylor a nice experience in a normal family environment. They didn't have a large home or lots of material possessions; instead they had each other, which was priceless. I never worried if I were running a little behind knowing Anjelina as well as her family were caring for him. There definitely was no better feeling for a mother than knowing your child was being well cared for and loved whenever you weren't around. I tried my best though to arrive every night by 6:30/6:35, after allowing myself 15 minutes of personal time to grab the mail at the post office and run to the grocery store.

The guilt forever lies in leaving Taylor for an entire day, and only seeing him for an hour or two at night, but it couldn't be helped. I was always there when push came to shove for meetings at school and the various doctors' appointments, but I had to do whatever it took to keep us afloat. Every day I got up in anticipation of being a caregiver and sole financial provider without the luxuries of another half to share the responsibility. If I went shopping it was with coupons clipped for the bare essentials or perusing with Taylor through the closeout racks for shoes and clothing for him. There definitely was no budget for a movie, manicure, or pedicure for myself let alone clothing. I made due with the few suits and clothes I had left from my single days, when I could work myself to death building my company, without having to worry about anyone else waiting for me at home.

Every once in a while, standing at the grocery store behind a typical family in our small suburban town with kids screaming in tow and a shopping cart overflowing with groceries for their one of two homes made me want to cry. We sure weren't taking weekend trips to Lake Tahoe skiing nor jetting off to Hawaii for winter break. I can't say I was ever resentful, just sad I couldn't do the same for Taylor, and sad I was all Taylor had at home. After five years, two surgeries for Taylor's ear tubes, countless doctors and therapist appointments, and no relief in sight, I was growing tired, and admittedly lonely. Then with a shrug, I learned to snap out of it and gather my strength and courage to see it all for what it was and look into my son's eyes. When he smiled and I heard his giggle, he always seemed to know exactly what I was thinking and we both laughed together. We have each other and we're as balanced as a two person family could be, and one of the happiest. It's all worth it.

After a small dinner party at my girlfriend's house, she insisted I try to start dating again. How in the world I would find the time I had no idea. Any spare time that I did have was spent just keeping up with work, eleven employees, researching new ways to help Taylor, and everyday housekeeping. Almost three years had passed though, and I admitted as well, maybe it was time, even if it was just someone to go to dinner with and have an adult conversation.

August 12, 2007, happened just as I had envisioned, Mr. Perfect came into my life. I had made a list of everything I wanted in a man, and he fit the mold with perfect proportions, minus one flaw that I never would have imagined, nor perhaps did I want to see: he was a United States Coast Guard Commander working at The White House and living full time in Washington, D.C. Our lives seemed to follow each other rhythmically for years yet never meeting. He was in Maine the same time I was. He lived in Healdsburg, CA the same time I was just forty miles away in my small suburban town, and his mother lived in Florida, my residence of thirteen years. Whenever I thought of him, he called. Whenever I reached into my mailbox wishing for a letter or card from him, it was there. I never in my entire life had such an intuition or connection with another person. He lavished me with expensive brief weekends in the wine country or for holiday skiing in Lake Tahoe when my mother could come stay at my home with Taylor. All trips that I could never financially afford to do as a single mother. His personality was so incredibly charismatic, intelligent and hysterically funny, you couldn't help but be in awe. I lived and breathed every text message and phone call just to hear his words of love, affection and kindness. Most of all, he wanted to settle down and start a family.

Every morning I woke him by a text at 2:30 a.m. from the West Coast to greet his day, or if he was on an assignment, he faithfully did the same. Countless poems, cards and small notes passed through my mailbox. He was my soldier hero at the beginning and end of every day, feeling as if I were Cinderella who had been waiting in anticipation for my knight in shining armor to save me. He was everything I had dreamed of in a human being. Compassionate, loving, extremely intelligent, always optimistic, handsome, and treated me like a princess. The miles never seemed to exist, and there was never any sense of time whether we were apart nor when we were together, it just felt as if time had stopped and we were one. It was an overwhelmingly serendipitous experience I had longed for. His gifts were perfectly executed and always extremely meaningful, like a Radio Flyer tricycle for Taylor's birthday or a special Lolia candle to light beside my bed for my morning coffee. A wonderful book of John Adam's love letters and cookbooks from our favorite restaurants throughout the country. Every note, or call or text came from his heart. Everything about him was beyond extraordinary and reached to my soul. He had worked amongst teams and as a leader under both the Clinton administration and later the Bush administration ensuring the President's safety, so surely he was of the utmost in trustworthiness for my son and me. The Coast Guard's moto: Semper Paratus. Always ready. And at the end of the day, the most important part of my life that was missing was someone I could trust with my heart and most especially my son's. And so it seemed, he was ready.

After months of courtship and his cross country trips to capture moments of time together, he was up for re-assignment with the Coast Guard one last time before he retired, and San Francisco was one of his potential new stations. Unbelievable! I had restructured my team at the showroom without having to remove anyone and brought us from number eleven in the country to number four behind New York, LA and Florida. Work was absolutely fantastic, and Taylor was well adjusted and having a blast in kindergarten. Everything was finally falling into place as I had prayed someday it would and I was finally getting a much needed personal break in my life, feeling invincible and on top of the world. On February 19th his orders came through and he was assigned to San Francisco. He would be the director of emergency response and operations covering the North West Coastline into Oregon. We were both elated as we would soon be together on a permanent basis. Or so I thought.

Taylor and I spent every weekend, researching and looking at properties in the beautiful and timeless wine region countryside. The idea was for us to keep my place in my suburban town for use during the week as he would be mostly at the Coast Guard Station at Yerba Buena Island just outside San Francisco. And for the weekends, the three of us would find a nice little wine country home. Every weekend Taylor and I would drive throughout the wine regions looking for the second house for us all and we'd search every corner of the wine country until we found it. In our search for a home, I found the greatest little BBQ restaurant in the tiny town of Glen Ellen. It was a two hundred year old grist mill with a huge waterwheel on the outside that Taylor loved to throw his Thomas the Trains into, not realizing they wouldn't come back to him! Taylor would stand in its' wake mesmerized by the spinning of the wheel and the water dripping from its notched troughs. Some would label the behavior as Autism, I just thought it was wonderful to see him enjoy something so simple that much. We'd look at properties all morning, then take a long hike in Jack London park with the tall lanky mossy green and grey trees overhanging the paved path, throwing rocks in the vast reservoir. The sun never seemed to stop shining in this almost mystical park, even when it was cloudy and grey with a slight mist of rain. We spent months combing the area looking for our perfect home with my Mr. Perfect and then savoring in the afternoon barbecued lunches of the old grist mill. Time seemed to stop whenever we were out there. The peace and quiet that surrounded us was intoxicating and Taylor and I were both at peace, together.

His arrival had finally come and the moving truck dropped his household contents into the final choice in a quaint little town surrounded by rolling hills of grape vines. It was the same home he had rented before he left on his second assignment back to The White House two years prior and he was absolutely thrilled. He had driven across country with his mother, and as the anticipation grew, so did his fears. I could hear it in his voice with every single phone call as he made the long journey. He was not only leaving a job he highly respected because his 2 years of duty had come to an end, but he was gaining a family at the same time. We spent a few days together over the weekend with his mother and slowly began unpacking his things into the home. She not only met Taylor, but couldn't have been more gracious or affectionate towards him, embracing him as if he were another grandchild.

The following Thursday afternoon, out of the clear blue, I was on a national managers conference call with eighteen people when I received a ping on my Blackberry. As I gazed down at the device that had brought me endless texts and e-mails of love and affection from my Mr. Perfect, I fell into a flushed faintness as I read the text ending our relationship. A cold, heartless text ended the hope I held onto for the past year of a normal life out of a *Town & Country* magazine publication with the man of my dreams. Within a mere 3 seconds my breath stopped and my body went limp and numb. My heart began to race and I feared what I was feeling were symptoms of a heart attack. I excused myself from the call, and told my staff I was ill and needed to leave immediately. I had never in my entire life had such a dramatic reaction to a situation. All sense of reason dissipated as I drove across the bridge and began to realize that I may possibly be having a heart attack. My chest felt like an elephant was sitting on it and my limbs were growing numb. Then I began to think of what a fool I was for driving myself the thirty odd miles to get home when I may in fact be having a heart attack. As I reached the rainbow painted tunnel just beyond the spans of the bridge, a snapshot of Taylor's bright smile flashed before my eyes creating a new focus. I needed to focus on that bright beautiful smile of his life and drive myself to the hospital. Focus and perseverance would bring me safely back home to my amazing son.

After being rushed through the E.R. and over three hours of tests, the doctor read through my test results and E.K.G. He consoled me; I wasn't having a heart attack, but rather an extreme panic attack. As the reality of the last several hours began to settle in, the vision I had had of my son's bright beautiful smile kept flashing through my mind. I was all he had and I needed to get it together because although I finally had a small life insurance policy, now was not the time to leave him. He needed me and I sure needed him, now more than ever. He was my rock, and without even knowing it at the time, I began to realize that he in fact may have saved my life for a second time from a man that didn't appreciate and respect both of us.

After several conversations with my former Mr. Perfect following this day, what I never even took into consideration in my blind love was another person not accepting my son for who he was as well as a mother for who she was. In my long list of conditions to describe the perfect man, I forgot the most important one: accept my son and me unconditionally, for the simple fact he is a child that has a disability and I am a very proud mother of my child.

It took almost a year to eat at our favorite barbecue spot in my fear of running into him and for the fond memories I still held on to. My heart will forever be broken not for a loss of a love, but the loss of hope. I lost hope in a portion of humanity that day and the hope I would have just a normal father for my son, and husband for me. The stares at the grocery store or the shopping mall were still there, and so were the lack of play date invitations. Our places of frequency were still minimal because of the ambient noises for Taylor and his sensory aversions to crowds as well as lots of commotion such as a simple baseball game. I was bound to isolation from a world that couldn't understand our world. My Mr. Perfect represented a world I no longer knew. I liked my new life with a perfectly imperfect child because it was real, it was tangible and open to failure. Mostly mine. For the first time in my life I didn't have to measure up to someone or something. I could be myself in Taylor's world and embrace my differences and faults just the same as his. Outside expectations and achievements were no longer so important to me. My hope instead turned to becoming a better person who could see the good in those around me, especially in the eyes of my son. My experience with Mr. Perfect really changed my life so unexpectedly, for once the heart ache of the loss dulled, I began to embrace Taylor and I's relationship like I had never done before. He really was my heart and soul, and I never wanted to disappoint him.

Taylor's world doesn't see cruelty. Everything that surrounds him is a world of play coming together as one big game. He doesn't have the burdens I see with most typical children. He's never angry and hardly ever cries or whines. Through Taylor, I began to see all of the amazing attributes of children who have disabilities. Their hearts seem so much bigger and their spirit seems so much wiser than typically developing children. Most of my observations were showing me how much more they seek love and acceptance from everyone, beyond anything I have ever seen in my forty years. Taylor's abilities of human compassion at six years old far outweighed his inabilities. I joke often with my close friends when I say, "Not liking Taylor is like not liking the Dalai Lama". Seriously. Taylor and every child I have ever seen that has Down syndrome is the most loving, social and charismatic person with a heart of gold. Their presence is such a gift to those that choose to see them for everything that they are. Their hearts and spirit are as gentle as the angels painted by the masters on the ceiling of Europe's basilicas. My son's world seems so exquisitely simple, peaceful and filled with kindness from the moment he wakes in the morning until he lays his head on his pillow at night.

My girlfriends and I remark a lot about how simple it was when we were children without all of the different social media sources, kids' activities and mindless television programs. We were all trying to apply some of our positive early childhood memories to our children's lives so they could remain the sweet innocent children we had once been, growing up without such high expectations. We were re-learning to try as best as possible to be home at 6:30 pm most nights so everyone could sit down to a nice meal, however big or small, and share in each other's day. We all agreed we were going to start by turning our Blackberry's and cell phones off and silence the television when everyone was together as a family. If we are able to set times for everything else in our day we figured, why can't we set one hour per day away for everyone to sit down together as a family when we could? Even if just to praise one another's accomplishments and embrace the time. My family sure wasn't the most functional when I was growing up, but we did sit down every night together and have an hour or so dinner. It created an air of stability and feeling of being a part of something as a unit. Under the economic duress many of us are experiencing, it's a mad scramble with schedules, both parents working, one parent home, the other at work. However, at the end of the day it really helps to know we're all in it together and just trying to provide the best life possible for one another. For me, it began and ended at home when I could actually be a role model for my son in positive ways. He would look at me for guidance, discipline, love, respect and acceptance and I needed to be all of that and more for him with more patience than I had never known I had.

I was also realizing when it came to Taylor and his various needs, I couldn't put the full responsibility on his school to "fix" him. It fundamentally had to start at home with me pre-teaching the skills I wanted to help him learn so he would eventually develop them on his own. I stopped myself often when I was about to send a scathing e-mail or call the school because they hadn't provided a tool or followed up on a previous request from me to help my son. It really wasn't their fault my son had a disability, and I surely can't expect them to "fix" everything. I began to understand my own personal stresses held within my sub-conscious could all too easily be vented on some poor helpless aide or teacher when in fact, I was just a frustrated parent frustrated at my own personal life and or set of circumstances I had never anticipated before the birth of my son. I needed to start many things at home first, and then ask the school to reinforce. And vice versa. I was learning every day how to adjust to my new world with a child that was different. I myself saw everything differently: family, friends, colleagues. The important wasn't so important any more, and I was more appreciative in being a part of Taylor's world.

A typical walk with Taylor is a veer off the sidewalk to peek in a hole in the bordering fence, and every time he does it, I have to laugh. He could care less we're about to be late for school and I needed to rush off to fight traffic to get to work. There might be something incredibly interesting in that hole in the fence. And so I stop, laugh and patiently guide him back onto the sidewalk. But what I am learning to do is take the time and look in the hole in the fence with him. When we do it together, it allows a mutual respect. Inevitably our eyes meet afterward, and we both burst out laughing. As the other parents hurriedly rush off panicking their child will be late to class, I quietly laugh and feel sad they don't stop with their own children and see why we're peeking in the hole in the fence. Instead they look at us with a silly expression, and continue past us barking at their little ducks in tow. Because of Taylor, I was growing up as an adult way beyond my years and loving everything he was so patiently teaching me.

CHAPTER 8

Patience

D ecember 18, 2008 I received a call from a wonderful job recruiter, Alison Moore. She knew that I was employed, but wanted to touch base and see if I was happy with the job. She was a very bright, hard-working single mother raising her son which gave us an instant bond.

The stresses at my job were increasing and the economy I could feel was about to shift. I have been in the luxury goods business long enough to know when to pull out and re-strategize before the market took me out on a financial level.

Alison said she had a very prestigious design firm in mind for me with a position they were trying to create, and all of my credentials were everything and more that they were looking for. Alison asked if I would at least consider taking a look at it and possibly interviewing with them. As I reflected throughout our conversation, my every day was spent worrying about finances and how Taylor and I were going to succeed. My own personal retirement was now put on the back burner because as a parent with a child of a disability, my new priority was to save for his retirement as well. I needed to remember to always think outside of the box for anything that may make our life easier and open to opportunity.

Never knowing if you were going to get the corporate axe regardless of how good you were was beginning to wear on me. Our showroom was doing extremely well, however, we were selling luxury goods. Hand blown Venetian glass from Murano, hand-woven textiles from mills around the world, and exclusive handmade furniture. There were always a variety of issues with shipping, quality, imperfections and it all fell on my shoulders. Prima donna designers didn't want to hear about a mill closing or an imperfect Venetian glass chandelier that was hand-blown, and not exactly the same as the one displayed in the showroom; especially given the extraordinary prices. They only cared that their product wasn't on time for installation, and on a daily basis, would either reach me on the phone and scream, or worse yet, they would come into the showroom and scream. It was a joke with my team that I had a turnaround time of three minutes or less, calming down even the most irate designer and finding a solution. You'd think their world was coming to an end because a piece of fabric was delayed a week. It's fabric people. Just fabric.

Anything beyond the care of a child almost dying at birth was almost silly and nonsensical to me. Nothing in life was more important than the health and wellness of a human being. It made my everyday working with the elite in any industry a piece of cake. I felt impervious to anything that came my way because I could rationalize the biggest of problems into the simplest within minutes. It was all about prioritizing and remembering what was really important first and dissecting the rest piece by piece for everyone else around me so they were all on the same page.

After months and years of looking out for so many people in my life, I began to re-structure my own life for Taylor and myself. Perhaps it was time for a change. Maybe a different job, better money and the chance to move my resume up one more notch was the right thing to do at this point. Working for one of the most prestigious and influential design firms on the West Coast would go far in my career experience. Perhaps I should at least listen to my recruiter friend Alison and her ideas on the job offer she wanted to present.

December 13, 2008 I met the owner of the infamous design firm for a cup of coffee in a beautiful little Italian coffee shop just a short distance from the renowned sailing boat docks in our neighboring town. I was so nervous, which was unusual for me, but I really needed to make a better life for Taylor and me and I knew just how much was at stake career wise if I decided to leave my cushy job managing the San Francisco design showroom.

The owner of the firm was incredibly articulate, sophisticated and, as an added bonus, we both had the same vision and understanding of design. I admit I prayed for a Christmas miracle, and just in time for the holiday, I had one. By the end of my cappuccino, I knew this change was the best choice for Taylor's and my future.

I stayed long enough managing the design showroom for the transition between the corporate office and the new manager as well as some construction we were doing. My new position would begin in January with the renowned designer and her thirty-eight person team on the exquisite Maiden Lane in San Francisco. I had no idea what I was doing, but I knew design, textiles and how to sell, so like everything else, I would figure it out.

I was still on the same schedule of dropping Taylor off at school and walking him into his class and then dashing into the city. The oatmeal was always embedded into the right shoulder of my suit from carrying him, but I learned in my flurry of the morning to now carry wet naps in my bag. In balancing the new commuting costs, I found an inexpensive parking lot four blocks from my new office for $6.00 per day if I got there before 9:00 a.m.. The coldest summer I ever spent was walking those four blocks. San Francisco is by far one of the most beautiful cities I have ever experienced, but it was amazing how cold it could be in the summertime!

The walking portion of my commute after leaving the parking lot, led me past the iconic Hermes, Gucci, Chanel and Christofle stores meticulously maintained with window washers polishing their fine glass panes every morning. Walking past the beauty within each and every stylized window was a designer's inspiration, because it held only the best of the best. It was also a constant reminder of my past when I could afford an Hermes scarf or a handmade pair of Donald Pliner shoes and I had to fight the feelings of envy when I saw someone my age walking out of the store with the bags I once held. I still didn't have a dime in my pocket to even walk in the front door and feel good about it, and even just to gaze within each store smelling the fine leathers and perfumes actually made me kind of sad. Especially when the retail staff were forever looking me up and down, pre-qualifying my wallet's potential before saying hello.

I peered in through the floor to ceiling windows laden with the latest trends thinking of my beautiful son and wanting to cry. I couldn't give him the luxuries of a life I once lived. Wishing I could walk in and buy something as simple as a silk scarf for me or a handmade little wooden train made in Italy I had seen for him. Something so luxurious that I could wrap around myself to sooth my weary mind and something so special for him he would forever cherish it. From the smells of freshly brewed cappuccino from the local barista, to the elegant people that shopped Maiden Lane—so beautiful and deliciously inviting, yet so far away from the realities of my new world. I was counting on this new job as my way to the ultimate in design success with more money, yet more expenses in commuting, more babysitters time . . . the vicious cycle just kept spinning. I had to get ahead.

As time went on I was traveling all over Europe, meeting with various textile mills for my new job, working around the clock with my mother flying back and forth from Southern California to San Francisco every time to watch Taylor while I was gone. I slept with my Blackberry and would always answer a call regardless if it were three in the morning to not miss the business lag in Italy, France or England.

I became obsessed with making more money to give Taylor better services, trying to balance our life at home and keep an eye on his education and medical needs. We were still attending horseback riding therapy for him on Saturdays and the rest of the week was its normal packed regimen of doctors and therapists along with school. Now I had to completely rely on the sitter, paying her more to shuttle him around while I traveled and worked late hours. I was becoming everything I didn't want to be without even realizing it because I was working so hard. I was becoming the career-obsessed mom that rarely saw her child, sacrificing my time with him for more money and financial opportunities. Even when we were together, I was so exhausted, I felt like I was barely functioning, and not being the quality mom I wanted and needed to be for him.

His kindergarten teacher was still amazing, as she always gave a phone call or sent a photo of his progresses while at school which helped my guilt complex. Also, knowing his babysitter Anjelina and her family were caring so well for him when I wasn't there eased my mind. But even with the extra support of Taylor at home and at school, I felt like a time bomb ready to explode and collapse. I was exhausted trying to keep up with everything seven days a week with no break in sight.

After eleven long arduous months, I exceeded every goal and challenge that was put in front of me in my new prestigious job. My responsibilities in the company were unattainable, but somehow, I made it successful. Being an overachiever comes at extremely high costs however. My health and general well being were compromised, and most of all, the time with my son. I was forever paranoid of losing my job for there was always a line of people that wanted it.

After traveling to the East Coast, Midwest and Southern California, I had closed the contracts for the representation of my designer boss's collections of luxury goods to be sold in Atlanta, San Francisco, Dallas, New York and Paris.

My own personal contract for commissions would finally begin with each sale adding to our monthly income. After months of anticipation and grueling long hours, I would fly to Paris just after the Christmas holiday to launch the first collection. It definitely was one of the most exciting times of my career. Until one day my worst fear came to fruition.

December 18, 2009 I was released from my position, forced to relinquish it to someone half the cost and half my age. As the words came out of the office manager's mouth, the room spun, my breath stopped and I remained in shock that cold December evening, and for months to come. I was rendered powerless once again. I gathered my bag and coat and made the long walk across the office. I never saw this coming, nor did our office manager as we both walked to the door. She, with humongous tears welling in her eyes. "I'm so sorry Kimberly" she said. "I had no idea." We hugged good-bye. Both of us were in complete shock that any employer could be so heartless and cold after I developed everything she would stamp her name on for years to come. All of my hard work was seen in every major Interior Design magazine throughout the United States and she collected all of the praise and acknowledgement when she did nothing more to the collections than tweak a color or two and make some simple design changes. The entire experience mirror imaged *"The Devil Wears Prada"* and the ruthlessness of the character Miranda Priestly.

I rode the elevator two floors down to the street below with twinkling lights embedded in the wreaths, trees and store front windows of Maiden Lane. It was a cold but beautiful clear night. The smells of the restaurants were wafting through the night air while hurried shoppers walked with their beautiful thick ribbon handled shopping bags. I was a single mom with no money that I was able to save beyond our everyday expenses, and I was lucky to be able to hock my car out of the garage to get home that night. Worse yet, it was a week before Christmas.

I was terribly crushed to be let go from a job I worked so hard at, sacrificed so much for yet, the fears of what lay ahead of us scared me even more. I had multiple offers the day after I was let go, so it wasn't too crazy, but nonetheless it was still a shock and complete blow to my ego. Re-focusing on what was in the best interest of my son and where I envisioned both of us to be in twenty years was my new mission. I also began to heal from the rejection of being let go of a life I was beginning to see as a past I never wanted to re-live again. I was relieved to have lost such an insanely exhausting job and so happy to go home to my son and get out of my suit. Far from this fake world that I no longer related to, washing my make up off and taking a hot bath, tossing my hair in a pony tail and throwing my jeans on. I had no idea what lay ahead, but I knew what I didn't want, and that was to feel this vulnerable and this afraid again in any future job that I had. I walked away knowing I not only did the best job I could possibly do, but it would be in every major design magazine for years to come for everyone to see, even if the credit went to the wrong person. I knew who really did all of the laborious work and I was proud of myself for it. And so, just like the ghost I became at my favorite barbecue restaurant in the wine country, I became a ghost in the design world. And now I could go home to my beautiful boy who would run to hug me the minute I got home, almost knocking me over. At the end of the day, I had faith in myself. I had to. My son needed me to.

The holidays were always tough as a single parent. As it is for any struggling parent with a family counting on you financially. I never had money enough for a lot of presents, and always made due with the hopes of a great Christmas bonus and the gifts from my friends and family for Taylor. The real joy was being able to spend the two weeks with him and the quality time that I had missed throughout the year. It was always a nice, quiet time of year without travel, and with lots of love from my little angel. Time was all I could really afford to give him and what I was truly beginning to see, was all he ever wanted from me in the first place. My time. He didn't care that we were completely broke, he just wanted to be with me. And what an honor that is for any parent.

After the holidays, I had to let the babysitter go because I now desperately needed the In Home Support Services financial resources we were getting instead of using it to pay her. So, I was back to the 24/7 week I had known before with Taylor. My best friend, Gavin, adamantly instructed me to go to the unemployment office and file an unemployment claim. I had no idea what any of it even meant, and I surely didn't know where to even begin. I'd heard of it before, but being self-employed, I never paid into unemployment prior to my last two salaried jobs nor did I ever need it.

The next day I packed Taylor up in the car and drove down to the unemployment office to see what I needed to do to file a claim. On arrival, with Taylor in his stroller, they told me children weren't allowed in the unemployment office. Funny. If I had a job, I could afford to pay the babysitter, and I wouldn't be here in the first place. "Shall I leave him in the hallway then?" I suggested wryly to the receptionist. The deeper I got into the local, state and federal offices and their bureaucracies, the more exhausted I became. And so, as Taylor and I remained in the hallway, they gave me the instructions to file so I could do it on my computer from home. Right . . . while my son was napping because I surely couldn't do it while he was awake! The humiliation grew.

I was trying to begin thinking outside of the box for whatever new job came my way, to be able to spend the quality time with Taylor that he needed. Freelancing in design wasn't going to work; I'd stepped away from my company for almost five years now and most of my contacts had moved on. And most things I was seeing on Craigslist or receiving referrals for were only paying minimum wage which wouldn't be close to an income sufficient to support one of us let alone two. So, I began survival mode once again until I had a solid offer with a new job that paid enough for our bills and the babysitter so I could work whatever hours I needed to.

As I researched all of our options, the doors were quickly closing. After my unemployment insurance income, we were still short the $1148.00 for my mortgage and the $436.00 for the condominium homeowners dues. I cut one expense after another trying to make ends meet. And then, as I was negotiating with the mortgage lender regarding my payment now due, she made a remark asking why I didn't file for a claim in the Job Loss Benefits Insurance program I had been paying into with my mortgage. Oh my gosh. I had no idea. By paying $100.00 per month more with my mortgage payment, I had bought myself up to 6 months time if I should ever lose my job. Within a few short weeks of filing the claim, they took over my mortgage payments saving our home, my credit rating and a great deal of personal humiliation. For as long as I live, I will forever pay into this. The same way I would always carry a good life insurance policy for Taylor. I just never knew what curve ball life was going to throw us.

I knew the food stamp program wasn't attainable. The maximum income for Taylor and me as a household of two was $1174.00 net per month and or $1579.00 gross per month. If my income was less than these figures, the maximum amount of food stamps for both of us for the entire month was $367.00. That breaks down to $6.11 per day per person for all three meals

Social Security Income or SSI, as it is known as for children with disabilities was the same situation. The maximum amount of allowed income for one parent with one child was $1640.00 per month and I was on the border line. Hence, this wasn't an option.

The WIC program was for mothers with infants under the age of five, and Taylor had just had his fifth birthday. So, this wasn't an option. The food bank was the only viable alternative for food and, somehow, I just couldn't make the trip again to the giant warehouse containing grocery store's random processed goods. Especially since Taylor's diet was so limited because of his oral aversions. For breakfast, he would only eat oatmeal I fortified with brown sugar and butter and Almond milk as he was allergic to regular milk. Snack was a vanilla La Creme by Dannon yogurt, and Gerber baby food bananas in a small 6 oz. jar. For lunch and dinner, he would only eat a special concoction of spaghetti I fortified with olive oil with sautéed and pureed fresh spinach mixed in with it. If you changed the noodle, or any of the taste and or consistency even in the slightest of any of his foods, he wouldn't eat it. The simple introduction of a new food made him gag and trying to switch the ingredients made him completely shut down and not eat anything at all.

Without funds to pay a specialist, I just couldn't move him past his oral aversions by myself. No matter how hard I tried. I love having this conversation with people. Have you tried ice cream, or cake, or french fries or mac and cheese? Have you tried real bananas or whip cream or . . . the list goes on. If a person has a hearing impairment, just because you speak louder, it doesn't mean they will be able to hear you. They are not able to hear, bottom line. The same goes in Taylor's case. I have tried every single piece of food in every kind of different way with him. Unless it is his normal known diet, he will not even try it. He may pick it up and throw it at you or on the floor, but he will not try it. The same problem extends to vitamins and medicines. He will not chew food, so why would he chew the oddly textured and unknown flavor of a vitamin? Hence, any medicine I give to him must be a (often sticky) liquid which I must shoot down his throat without him aspirating via a small plastic syringe.

As an odd side thought that was always lingering in the back of my mind, what would I do if California finally had the major earthquake they were always talking about? I can muscle through an earthquake, but I can't muscle through Taylor's finicky diet without a proper back up plan, just in case the day did come when I had to deal with a natural catastrophe. A large bin of diapers, Pediasure, and the non-perishable portion of his diet were always set aside just in case along with the camp stove with propane to cook his spaghetti. I figured out the things that would sustain him like his Pediasure that's packed with most of what he needed nutritionally for a full day. And if I'm traveling with Taylor, it's a life saver because he normally doesn't acclimate very well to new surroundings when on the go, and he definitely wouldn't eat his regular food if he's not completely comfortable with his environment.

Taylor's hearing along with his food aversions was another issue to contend with. After six years of testing, doctor's appointments and speech therapies, we now faced the reality that Taylor's hearing was still reading at the mid-range level. After two tests per year between UCSF (University of California San Francisco) and the Speech and Hearing Institute, we were finally given the go ahead at his school to have an FM device put into Taylor's classroom so he could better hear what the teacher was saying. It's a small speaker in a prominent place within the classroom, and the teacher is given a small microphone to speak into. They also requested a closer spot within the classroom to the teacher for his hearing impairment.

I'd been trying desperately to have a speech and feeding assessment done in light of the hearing loss as they are basically one assessment. They would also do a behavioral evaluation so everything could be tied in together with regards to therapy.

Taylor still didn't have one word he was able to speak and with his lack of hearing the words clearly, as well as their enunciation, it was difficult to say how long it would be before he would speak. As a part of the same evaluation, we could tie in his oral aversions which directly and indirectly correlate with his speech. I had finally found the specialists all under one roof at CPMC (California Pacific Medical Center Child Development Center) in San Francisco. We had a direct referral by the Speech and Hearing Institute, however his Medi-Cal Insurance wouldn't pay because it didn't fall under their plan with regards to allowed specialists. And even if it were gifted by a relative or private organization, it would then fall against the policies of Medi-Cal, so I couldn't ask relatives to help pay for it.

I tried CCS (California Children's Services) and they couldn't authorize it either. Now mind you, I really don't mind researching more, and playing mom turned doctor—therapist—psychologist—researcher, but I have absolutely no medical or psychological experience nor book references to even know where to begin with all of this. I was just a mom looking to give the basic needs to her child. So, the medical professionals all directed me back to the public school my son was at to put the onus on them to provide more speech within the classroom and/or more one-on-one in a "pull out" session. Therefore, the process started all over again to call another meeting at his school to implement and advocate for more speech in the classroom and more speech time with his therapist thru his IEP. The days, weeks and months continued to go by as we filled out the paperwork, scheduled meetings and discussed the implementation of the FM device and more speech. However, we still had no one qualified to work on his feeding therapy which directly correlated to his speech issues. And, this still didn't help the behavioral aspects of feeding, speech and his challenge with varying environments.

Day after day, the struggles in a system I had no idea how to navigate became more and more challenging and frustrating. And I was one of the lucky ones who didn't have to deal with issues like feeding tubes, wheelchairs, and heavy amounts of medication. The medical costs were becoming increasingly unattainable, even with the smallest of prescriptions. Taylor's need for medicine to help with his acid reflux, out of the blue, was no longer covered under his Medi-Cal insurance. Doctor's visit co-pays had recently increased and the majority of his therapies were no longer covered under any portion of any of the state services or insurance. As the legislators within our state bickered and negotiated what nine billion dollars in programs would be cut, they included those very same programs that I had diligently paid into as hard working tax paying U.S. Citizen.

Without the proper funds for private insurance (which didn't cover many of our health needs anyway) my son was unable to get the basic needs in healthcare. The same went for his education. So many of our Congressmen and politicians passing reforms to programs in my son's education and healthcare would only hurt him in the long run and deny his very access to a better education and quality of life. However, when it came to their own children, I'm sure they were in private schools and could afford private health insurance, thanks to our support of their extraordinary paychecks and benefits. They weren't personally affected by their own actions or inactions. I often wondered for all of those passing such severe financial cuts, how many of them also had a child with a disability. What was their reference and experience in knowing what our children with special needs or disabilities really needed?

CHAPTER 9

Independence

The minute I told relatives and a couple of select friends I had lost my job, the flurry of their expectations rose to the surface of our conversation once again. What are you going to do? How are you going to live, pay your mortgage and buy food? What jobs are you going to apply for? You need to get a recruiter tomorrow. Surf Craigslist. Get out there and comb the newspaper want ads. Knock on doors. Talk to people. Have you even begun to look for work? Did you file for unemployment yet? The comments kept coming. Just the same as after Taylor's birth. I was expected to swallow my grievances, get a job, and find a way to support both of us within weeks of his birth and diagnosis. What kind of super human powers does everyone think that I have? Do they not think that I know all of these things? I think everyone just got used to me always picking myself up in the hardest of times and held the same high expectations whenever I did fall. Instead, I really just needed a shoulder to cry on and someone to listen to our challenges and concerns.

Those who were trying to help had never experienced the specialness of a household with a child who had special needs. I hadn't either, but I sure lived it every day. Only my best friend Joe and my Florida family were actually asking me what I needed. Whether it be a toy, or clothing or some kind of self-help book for Taylor's special needs. When Uncle Joe heard we were having problems with Taylor's communication, he sent us every single DVD on sign language called *"Signing Times"* by Two Little Hands Productions. Uncle Joe researched and sent countless books on Down syndrome, feeding skills, and communication skills after hearing my frustrations on each subject. When it was a holiday or Taylor's birthday, Joe and my Florida family were always there with a meaningful gift. When it was back to school time, they sent all of Taylor's clothing so he was always prepared. But not without always asking what Taylor's real basic needs were first. Our condo was only 756 square feet, and there wasn't a lot of room for anything but the necessities.

I think the biggest problem with family is that they wanted to help for the most part, they just didn't know how. My family projected their thoughts, feelings and own parenting skills onto me without actually ever listening. I was increasingly becoming overwhelmed by feelings of resentment, anger and complete frustration with how I was expected to raise my son. It became a vicious cycle, and even more exhausting because my son needed so much of me already. I really didn't need more with relatives telling me how to raise him. I had enough going on every day without the drama of any outside parties.

At the end of the day, I am the parent and it was my home. My decisions may not always be spot on, but, I am the one caring for my child every single day no matter how difficult the caregiving is. I am the one living at the hospitals and doctors and therapists offices day in and day out. I need to be respected, honored, and loved just as any other parent. My decisions for my son should be respected, and my own opinions and beliefs needed to be honored regardless of what others do within their own homes. I may not always be correct with my approaches to Taylor's needs, but I do know how much research I normally do for even the slightest change in his diet, communication and health care, often times, knowing a little more than some of his doctors, for the simple fact I live it every day and experienced it firsthand. As my son's parent, I was the expert and it needed to be respected.

I have been at fault for allowing my own mother to cross the parent line. I allowed her to tell me what to do, where to go and when out of sheer exhaustion. My son's birthday parties, holidays and outings were all chosen by my mother, and if I didn't follow suit the amount of guilt that came with it wasn't worth the confrontation. I allowed her to control my own feelings about things because it was easier, and I never liked confrontations after dealing with my ex-husband. I learned a long time ago it was always best to just remain quiet and walk away rather than confront someone. At no one else's fault but my own. I wasn't taking the fifteen minutes to take a walk after I dropped Taylor off at school. I was no longer going to the gym, and for the first time in years sometimes I wouldn't shower or dress outside of my sweats. I couldn't even remember if I had brushed my teeth that morning. I had to change.

I'm not too sure what the catalyst was, but shortly before my forty-first birthday I woke up early one morning, grabbed a steaming hot cup of coffee, and watched Taylor sleeping like a little angel tucked away in his bed. A wave of emotions flooded my mind and body and I knew I had to be the change for him. I felt the sensation of just finishing college and feeling that the world was at my door step waiting for me to experience it like never before. The world was mine to live, love and explore, only this time through the eyes of my son. I had had enough, and no one could tell me different, because I removed myself from their expectations and judgments. At forty-one years old, just as I had allowed myself at twenty-four, I took control of my life again and allowed myself to cry, run, or take a few hours off to climb a local mountain. All I wanted was the peaceful silence I was trying to find again in my own mind, just as Taylor lived every day. I aspired to be more like him now. I began to listen to music in my car after I dropped Taylor off at school so loudly the doors shook. I rolled down the windows and opened the sun roof, cranked up the stereo and drove onto the highway with no place in particular as a destination. The destination was me.

When I picked Taylor up at school four and half hours later, I kept the windows down, lowered the music to his level, and we both danced. The smile in the back seat was as big as a football field. We were becoming everything I had hoped. A team. I may not be able to be his best friend in life, but I will always be his mother with complete unconditional love and respect. Respect for everything that he is, and appreciation for those things he may not be. I needed to be a mom first, not his multiple therapists, advocate, or behaviorist, but his mother before anything else. It was an extremely powerful, joyful and yet sorrowful time, as it did mean letting some people go. Those that didn't empower me or Taylor would have to take a step back.

Taylor's energy level was that of a typical toddler and his interests were expanding, which was so fantastic developmentally for him! However, at the same time he was now also requiring some pretty extreme additional time to harness the energy and make it a beneficial experience for him. As I worked on my parenting skills, and redefining our lives to better Taylor's in the longer term, I was meeting new challenges on the home front with regards to his behaviors. He was becoming increasingly agitated (and I couldn't blame him) because he still didn't have words he was able to speak, nor the ability to sign. His different noises all have a purpose to him and yet he just couldn't formulate the words to give them meaning to me. Now, we both do the best we can to communicate in more non-conventional ways.

For example, if he wants a DVD to watch, he tugs on my hand until I stop whatever I'm doing and guides me to the kitchen, points to the top of the fridge which is where I keep the DVD case and won't let go of my hand until I take it down for him. His fine and gross motor skills had advanced enough now where he could actually unzip the case, choose his DVD and turn the television on and control all of the buttons to play it. Something so simple to others is a huge step in our house. Not that his learning to turn the TV on for himself is always a good thing, but it's all about compromising! The key when it is just the two of us is independence. And, for his future life building skills, it's all about having the patience, taking the time and showing him how to do everything step by step. With him, it may take a few more times than one of his peers but he gets it eventually. And when he does, I praise him like there is no tomorrow, and as I do, he beams from ear to ear over his accomplishment. Validation became a driving force in how I raised him and slowly built his confidence.

On the flip side, if he doesn't get what he wants, he'll quite simply just drop to the floor and cry. It doesn't matter if it's the middle of the parking lot or grocery store, just as I used to do when I was a little girl. He stops and drops and won't move until you physically stop everything and pick him up. I can't obviously allow him to get or do everything he wants, but I can stop, drop to his level and tell him that. I hug him and say, "No. I'm sorry baby, you can't just run in the street or a car will hit you. But, why don't we go to the park so you can run there." Or, "No. You can't play with the trains now, but you can bring a train with you because we need to go to the store." I offered him the recognition of his need, the acceptance and acknowledgment of his desire, and then an alternative plan so he felt validated. If I spoke too sternly or loudly, you could see him withdraw back into himself and shut down in front of your eyes. Times like these, I wondered just how much the domestic violence affected him while he was in the womb. I was becoming more and more aware of his nuances, and was slowly adjusting our lives to compensate for them. It was easier and much less exhausting for me to do this than it was for me to try and force him to adjust to his surroundings sometimes.

This was one area I was realizing was much different when working with a child of any intellectual or developmental disability. I had seen children over the years in the grocery store or the shopping mall having a meltdown because they didn't get what they wanted, and I always bit my tongue when the parent didn't do anything about it. Now I was beginning to see another side of the equation. Was the child I was observing in the grocery store or mall a typical child just having a meltdown or was it a child that appeared to be a typical child, yet had Autism or another neurological disorder? I began to build my tolerances and let go of judgments because it may in fact not be a parent that is negligent in their parenting, but a parent that is digging through the behavioral trenches of a child with an intellectual or developmental disability.

I was in a Baby Gap a couple of years ago waiting patiently in line behind two women purchasing their items with their children. One of the little boys began to kick the other woman's child for no apparent reason. As he was a stranger to the little girl, and the fact that the kicking was probably really hurting her, she began helplessly crying. The scene of kicking and crying between the two children continued for almost five minutes. I finally looked at both mothers and, in a very calm and rational voice, acknowledged for them that the little girl was being kicked in hopes the kicking parties' mother would correct the situation. Instead, the mother quickly turned on her heels and glared at me sharply, stating I didn't know what I was talking about. I quietly and confidently replied, yes I do. I am the proud mother of a child with an intellectual disability with his own behavioral issues, and it's called discipline; I retracted eloquently but sharply. A typically developing child's discipline is pretty straight forward and a bit easier to measure and predict. However, at least I can speak on behalf my son with Down syndrome, the techniques used in his discipline need to be modified so he has the time to process the situation. A softer, non-yelling and certainly non-hitting approach became a much better asset in getting the results needed. He just would never understand the spank on the bottom the same way, nor would he understand someone yelling at him. Taylor on the few times I have raised my voice to him will look straight at me and laugh or just completely melt to the floor crying uncontrollably. The synapse connection was much slower, and so I learned to discipline as I stated previously by showing love and validation. It worked so much better and I was able to get a faster correction to the negative behavior. A small moment in time was given to him so he could understand why I was upset or a privilege was taken away and well explained as to why it was taken away. As one very special parent said to me once "Try to pre-teach the skills or behaviors you would like to see. Pre-teaching is very often a much better, proactive way to teach any child let alone a child with any neurological issue." Leading by example, and teaching my son first the behaviors I wanted to see followed by repetition gave us both a more even playing field in understanding each other.

There also seems to be a very large grey area when it comes to the behaviors and disciplining of children with special needs as far as the classroom is concerned. I have heard nightmare stories of children with special needs being sent to the principal's office or even suspended for their negative behavior. Within at least our Down syndrome community (as this is my dominant resource) a negative behavior often arises as the result of poor team planning and management within the classroom environment. My son is an extremely kind, social and completely non-aggressive child unless another child instigates. If he is constantly bullied or another child is bothering him, he will push back in one way or another. Without the speech to defend himself, I always hoped someone within the classroom would see what was happening, otherwise it could be misconstrued as Taylor being the aggressor.

As Taylor goes through his regular general education schooling with a well planned and organized team to support him, I run into those parents whose children have stayed in a special education school. More often than not, the child has become much more aggressive, throwing toys, hitting, biting and acting out not only at school but at home, because they are forced to be around only children with intellectual and developmental disabilities and not around typically developing children. They model the negative behaviors due to the frustrations in their communication, peer interaction or, often times, the sheer lack of teachers or aides. Within a general education classroom, if all children are fully included (depending again case by case) they observe on a daily basis how the majority of society acts and also reacts to situations. If they are bad, and their behavior is unacceptable, it is the responsibility of the teacher and the aide to understand the cause first, and then alter the situation so the child with the disability understands the negative behavior, and is taught how to avoid repeating the behavior. Sending the child to the principal's office or removing the child from the class and isolating them in a special education room doesn't solve the problem but increases misunderstanding of the situation for the child.

In all of my research and interviews with parents and educators alike, a lot of the problem was the lack of training for teachers and aides with children of varying disabilities. Without having the support and training of a strong general education and special education inclusion team, the general education teacher (mostly those without enough training or experience with special needs) simply won't know what to do if certain problems arise as well as their ability to effectively teach the entire classroom inclusively. Rather than speak up and question, out of pride and ignorance perhaps, they may blame the issue on the child, removing them altogether from the classroom. It's a complete lose—lose situation.

Parents like me were finding more supports needed to be implemented in our children's classrooms to deal with the socioeconomic implications, cultural differences, learning disabilities, and language barriers of all children. Whether a child without a disability needs a little more time and assistance in taking a test or another child needs more support because English is his or her second language, I wanted to know how and what tools needed to be implemented so they could fully participate and learn within their classroom. I was truly beginning to worry that the problems in our schools may only increase with our current environmental and global financial crises as well as a rising number of children with disabilities. When I began understanding my son's world and reading the statistics, there was a 1 to 166 ratio of children that were being diagnosed with Autism. This year, I just read it has dramatically increased to 1 in 88 children are being diagnosed with Autism. I don't want to look back on my life and think I didn't help families and their children with disabilities after living it every day. It wasn't just about my son, but all families and all children that were going through the same pains and experiences. All of my years of research taught me that most children with disabilities (of course there are always exceptions) could be included in regular general education classroom amongst their typically developing peers. With a little classroom preparation and teacher guidance, they could participate equally.

I have great hope for our educational system and the spirit that lives within so many incredible teachers that truly want to make a difference in our children's lives. However, someone must begin to bridge the gaps between special education and general education and lower the hurdle not only for educators, but also the children themselves. I see my son and all children as our future and the investment in them may be the only certainty we have for a better quality of life and community experience.

CHAPTER 10

Life Beyond the Label

Every night after dinner, Taylor and I walked around our pristine suburban neighborhood to talk with neighbors and say hello to fellow walkers. With the slight slant of Taylor's eyes, and his occasional verbal utterance's, I would watch the expressions on some fellow walker's faces as they stared at Taylor as if I'm not even there. Rather than saying hello to him or me, and making brief recognition of the difference and pushing past it in a fleeting moment, they chose to ignore us. The pain in my heart deepened from the lack of respect for my son, and then the protective mothering instinct emerged, readying me to pounce like a great thundering mountain lion on them should they say anything negative. Yes my son is a little different, and he makes some funny noises because he doesn't talk yet, but he's a really cool kiddo if they would just get to know him. And yes, my son really likes to stop and look in every single drain in the neighborhood because there might be something extremely exciting in one of them.

So as people stare and make their snide comments, instead of my replying with the same, I have learned to give a very happy smile and greet them to something positive. "Hi. Beautiful day isn't it? Yep, he sure loves those drains! Just a typical boy!" Just as I give Taylor validation, I acknowledge their misunderstandings about him by making it approachable for them as a normalcy rather than a difference. I reached inside for the person I aspired to be and made it a positive moment. I used to think I was trying to do it for Taylor, however now I recognize I'm doing it more for the community so everyone feels comfortable and accepted.

I felt I could be the better person here, and lead by example in accepting everyone for who and what he or she is, regardless of differences. I was noticing that people's curiosity about him and children like him could be misconstrued as judgmental or as an ignorant stare. But maybe, just maybe, before Taylor was born I stared in curiosity when I saw someone that was obviously different from me. Regardless, I wanted to treat others as I wanted to be treated.

For example, one evening, Taylor and I walked our same loop in the neighborhood when a very nice father of two toddlers introduced himself and asked, "Where do I recognize you from?"

"I'm not sure," I replied. "Perhaps the elementary school?" I asked.

"No, no." he replied. "I had seen a group of "Them" at Bumble and Bumble preschool, and thought I saw your son there."

Now, as I froze in my spot on the concrete sidewalk, not quite believing this man just labeled my son and a small group of children with disabilities, as "Them" I stopped myself from completely bashing his ignorance, because my reality is not his. And quite frankly, I can't force my beliefs of everyone living in my utopian, "My son is like everyone else" kind of world. My son is seen differently in the greater whole of society and I cannot change that, nor do I want to force it on someone. I love him for everything that he is, and often times wish others would change with regards to respecting people with obvious differences, but I can't. However, what I can do is mentor a school of thought and social paradigm to help people understand Taylor as a person first and a disability second. I found a great group trying to bring awareness to this school of thought called People First.

And so now I am finally getting the courage to have better replies when someone says something which comes across in my heart as a judgment or ignorance. As in the instance with this particular father, I kindly replied, "Oh, you mean my son Taylor, who has Down syndrome? No, actually he is in the same general education school as your daughter just down the street. Perhaps that is where you recognized us from?" So what I have done here is not transfer my anger, but taught him Taylor is a person first. Disability second. It may resonate in this father's future dialogue, it may not, but at least I can be at peace with knowing I advocated for my son and helped to break down one more barrier.

At our local grocery store, there was a wonderful older woman that took care of the grocery bagging. For four years, she kept asking me every single time I was in the line with Taylor, "Is he talking yet?" Every single time could be up to five times per week. Now, I realize this is a sore spot for me in the first place because Taylor still wasn't uttering his first word, but eventually I found myself moving to a different cashier and line whenever I saw her because I couldn't stand to hear the words one more time. And now, after re-analyzing the situation, I realized it was my problem. First, it was my problem that I didn't acknowledge to myself that it was a personal frustration my son wasn't speaking yet, and secondly, that she had a small intellectual disability herself that wasn't completely obvious when speaking to her in those brief moments going through the checkout line. I was so in my own world rushing through the store, I didn't validate her innocent thoughts or concerns about my son. I was so conditioned to always be on guard, ready to pounce like a mountain lion. She was really in her own quirky way trying to be encouraging. She wanted to talk to him, and get a response, but she knew he couldn't and I think it really bothered her. Hence, the asking every time if he could talk yet. Maybe she really just wanted him to validate her.

Taylor's biannual Medi-Cal "well-being" checkup included a blood sample at UCSF's children's hospital in the city. Upon arrival, we were instructed to go to a small room in the 200 Building on Parnasis Street on the second floor. As we sat patiently in the tiny waiting room, a woman and her son arrived to have his blood drawn. Within moments of their arrival, it was clear he was not happy to be there and just wanted out. He was a very highly functioning child around thirteen years old, yet had quite an apparent intellectual disability. Taylor was happy just hanging out and playing, so I asked them to go in first to have the boy's blood drawn, to avoid any more distress for him and his mother.

A few minutes later, they emerged from the blood drawing room, and the mother kindly told her son she needed to use the restroom. She instructed him to sit and wait for her just outside the door and that she would be right out and then they could go home. He followed the direction clearly and with an almost childlike enthusiasm, sat next to me. Within a minute of the bathroom door closing, he looked at me, then my handbag and proceeded to open it. To me, it was a violation and invasion of my personal space, but to him, it was perhaps a small treasure trove of goodies that he just wanted to explore. As I gently said, "No, please don't do that," he became terribly sad and just got up and walked away. He walked away because instead of me validating him and giving him an alternative, I had said "no" directly without an option. Perhaps in his mind, it was too difficult of a concept to a process, filter and understand and therefore he would rather avoid the confrontation, just as Taylor would have done and walked away.

I followed him with Taylor and we eventually guided him back until his mother came out of the bathroom, but it taught me that perhaps in his own way, he had given me an opportunity to interact with him and because it wasn't a verbal request from him, I misinterpreted his actions, wants and needs. He was clearly a very capable and intelligent person that just couldn't communicate the same as most people could. He was a person first, disability second.

It has taken me six years to fully understand the real meaning behind the concept of "people first" when I interacted with families and their children with whom have disabilities. Since my son's birth, at the hospital, doctors' offices and even the paperwork at the schools, all of his paperwork is all written with the diagnosis as "mentally retarded." Even in the most recent meeting with his school psychologist, she referenced several times to the written words mentally retarded in his psychological evaluation. The words impaled my heart every time someone used them directly or indirectly when referring to my son. It's such a raw, derogatory word. Retarded. It's brash, demeaning and demoralizing, and thankfully, others are recognizing its inappropriateness as well.

On Tuesday, October 5, 2010, President Barack Obama signed into law S. 2781, "Rosa's Law," which changes references in many Federal statutes that currently refer to "mental retardation" to refer, instead, to "intellectual disability". The family of Rosa Marcellino, a nine year-old girl with Down syndrome, worked with their state representative to pass the legislation in the Maryland General Assembly. Rosa's Law is about families fighting for the respect and dignity of their loved ones. It is a great accomplishment by a wonderful little girl, something that she has passed on to every child in the future. She and her family should be proud of themselves for this accomplishment. We may not be able to change everyone, but we may, one by one be able to inspire the change we want to see in the world.

As I spent more time around Taylor's fellow friends and our Down syndrome support group, I began to understand the importance of language when referring to him and his friends as well as how important it was to be his advocate in our everyday life. It's never easy. Often times I would rather stay within the safe shelter of our own home, harboring my son from a world that may not understand his diversity. But I also realize just how important it is to get Taylor out into the community as much as possible for him, for me, as well as the rest of the community because just being present and being as "normal" of a family as possible creates its own awareness and hopes for eventual acceptance. I'm not sure what normal really means anymore, but I do know Taylor and I as a family are completely "normal" until I step out my front door. And I have to laugh, because I have never seen so many un-normal people in my life than within my small suburban community of San Francisco. Our town and surrounding area is one of the most beautiful places I have ever lived, however, the "typically" developing children that are surrounding us aren't so perfect, and neither are their parents because they don't have the compassion to see my son as a valued community member and as their child's peer.

Inclusion isn't just a philosophy within a school, it had to be a philosophy throughout the community and I knew with enough research I would find that very same community for my son. When families don't have the experience or exposure to children with disabilities, I thought, well of course they don't understand our world, they had never experienced it before. More and more I began to see the need to help all parents bridge the gap between typically developing children and those with disabilities. This period of time in my son's life was easy because he was only in kindergarten amongst children with new inexperienced minds. As he grew into his adolescent and teenage years, that gap would become much greater as he realized how different he may be from his peers if they didn't accept him.

Our time in our small California town was limited with respect to Taylor's future needs. Financially, the budget cuts to education, services and Medi-Cal had us on a time clock to move out of the state because it just was becoming so impossible to make a decent living and afford the taxes and high costs of living as a single parent. It was too expensive no matter what I tried. It became a never ending cycle of socioeconomic implications when they started cutting an already broken educational system, and with the housing crisis, it would probably only get worse for parents like me and children like Taylor. Besides, through my tireless research, it looked like Taylor would be much better off in the northeastern region of the United States where inclusion is a way of life in the schools and within the communities.

I yearned for a more balanced, accepting and forward thinking community, and yet until then, I was absorbing every piece of knowledge possible with regards to what wasn't working in our community and others like it, so maybe someday I could go back and teach them to build a stronger community and help try to make a difference for those that didn't have a voice. Both in our current community and throughout the country! I wanted to help our new world of people with disabilities grasp life's possibilities not life's limitations. Due to Taylor's cognitive age level, size and abilities, we kept him back another year in kindergarten. This step bought me a little more time—an added bonus on the home front and time to figure out where we could move.

With the new year, and the new budget cuts, it also brought a new team to our elementary school and of course a different kindergarten teacher than the one Taylor had progressed so well with. Change is never easy for Taylor, nor myself where he was concerned. Once the classroom door closes, I have no idea how he is unless the teacher calls or e-mails because my son is non-verbal. The teacher and aide are my life lines, and if that one-on-one communication isn't there, I am steering completely blind.

Our team for Inclusion at the school entails a Special Education Coordinator, a Special Education Teacher, Occupational Therapist, Speech and Language Therapist, and an aide. The previous year we had the most perfect team, all working rhythmically together and always including me as a team member. Our superintendent did an excellent job in hiring the previous Special Education Coordinator Stephanie Simms who had saved Taylor from the "disabilities only" preschool.

However, the new team brought change at a time that I wasn't prepared for and neither was Taylor. The prior year's team made everything run so smoothly and Taylor had a banner year. They always anticipated his needs and promoted his strengths while recognizing his weaknesses and bolstering him so he could succeed within each weakness. However, with the new team came an apparent lack of experience, training and care in including Taylor and those like him. It would soon create a rift between the parents and the faculty as well as an animosity toward an ill-functioning system that now all of a sudden was no longer able to hide. Under this perfect storm, everything that wasn't working at the school would come to the surface and become ever more transparent.

The teachers and aides had been instructed by the new Special Education teacher to funnel all requests by any parent through her.

Additionally if they had any information, it needed to go through her first; she would filter the information, and only until that happened could it be acknowledged and dealt with. Everything was being controlled by a brand new, fresh out of school teacher with almost no experience in dealing with children like my son. All of the valuable information that used to flow between all of us in our prior team was now being controlled and not shared, only hindering my son's every day school experience. Taylor was now running out of the classroom, hiding under the tables and without the structural support and direction from the teacher, there was no hope in sight for him to access a proper education. Within just a few short months, he had regressed dramatically, and regardless of how many meetings I called, it was beyond my ability and for that matter, responsibility.

From my beginning days in college, to my years of building teams within my company, all great creativity began through a series of thumbnails. The series depicted sometimes hundreds of scenarios and visions for the outcome we wanted to see and the changes that could be implemented if designed well enough. It was a fabulous collaboration of efforts by all designers and was fueled by intense creativity, imagination, experience and most importantly, team work. In my experience, trying to control my team too tightly only hampered a successful result. Communication between the teacher, therapists, aide and parent were absolutely critical in the development and success of each individual child and the situation wasn't really any different than the collaborations and team work I once directed in my company.

And so, I tried to guide my way through on Taylor's behalf without overstepping my boundaries as a parent. If my son was not getting what he needed in accommodations and didn't have the proper tools to access his education, someone had to step in and intervene, regardless of how exhausting or frustrating it was for me. I couldn't help thinking this just shouldn't be my job or any parents for that matter. This wasn't my formal training. Yet the inexperience of just one new teacher had a ripple effect and halted the progress of the most important component: the child.

I learned to gravitate towards the couple of teachers from the previous year and honed in on them and their skills and talents with Taylor, sometimes sidestepping the "correct process" so I could get the extra speech therapy he needed or some tips on feeding skills from his speech therapist. I learned to only communicate directly with the therapists, teacher and aide and ignore the Special Education Director and Special Education Teacher. If they weren't willing to be on a team, acting as a team member, then I had no use for them. Whatever it took, I just wanted my son to succeed, and I was learning to work around the system rather than trying to constantly battle it. It had been taking a toll on my health and I recognized it. Sleepless nights worrying he wasn't getting the services we had carefully mapped out in last year's IEP, or worrying over the fact Taylor hadn't been asked to one play date or birthday party throughout the year.

As of June 2010 we were supposed to have the Additional Assessment for an Alternative Augmentative Communication device done, and it was now December. (An Alternative Augmentative Communication device is a fancy term for a voice output system in which the child has a small device with several icons or words on it. The child pushes the button with the want or need or word they want to speak and it speaks for them. There is also a wonderful new device by Dynavox called the *EyeMax System* in which the child with mobility issues can just look with their eyes at the word or icon and select it through their eye movement). We were still waiting behind the sixty others that had requested the same thing or similar. There were too many children in need of additional help, little staff to support it, and it was even worse on the county levels where the children were still segregated into Special Education classrooms. There was even talk of further consolidation between the county and district schools, combining all children, yet they weren't providing the basic infrastructure to support it like trained and qualified Special Education Teachers and enough General Education Teachers. We were finding many of the General Education Teachers throughout our school and the outlying areas weren't properly trained to understand and teach children who were English Language Learners, children with disabilities or even children with cultural differences, nor did many of them want to. Many of them were tenured into the system and not required to have a Special Education, ELL background or training to handle cultural diversity.

I began to take more of my son's education back into our home and work with him more on my own, not only with his life skills, but with his overall education. I created picture schedules on the front door at home depicting six different outdoor activities and or places. Horseback riding, car, walk, store, biking, and playground. Whenever we went somewhere, I had him point to the icon so he knew where were going, or, it gave him a choice of picking where he wanted to go. I did the same thing with our refrigerator. He has each of his foods individually photographed and Velcroed to the fridge so anytime he wanted something to eat or drink, all he had to do was pull it off the fridge and give it to me. Until he had words, it was the best communication system between us. I kept trying sign language with him, but without it being reinforced at school, it was a one way street.

Our best times were reading books and the game *Starfall* on the computer. When I asked his speech teacher to see what else we could start doing to increase his speech and language, she began to show me the school's new IPad Touch and pulled up the program *Starfall* on the screen for Taylor to demonstrate. I'd been playing it on my lap top and he had to point to each word and then I'd press the key pad or helped him to do the same. With the IPad Touch, he controlled every single letter with his own hand, and even placed all of the shapes in the correct spaces when asked to do so. As the letter 'M' came up, it said the sound, "MMMM" and Taylor simultaneously mimicked it! I was in shock. I had experienced a little of his accomplishments at home on my computer, but not to the full extent that the IPad allowed, mostly because I think he knew he was in charge. It was his game that he could successfully manipulate all by himself and he was enthusiastic to keep trying it over and over again. In times like these, it was absolutely fantastic to see as a parent just how much he could do given the right tools, guidance and teaching, and I was grateful to his incredibly talented and dedicated speech therapist, Claire Shanahan. She broke down Taylor's barriers and truly got to know him, often spending countless hours outside of the classroom working with him and building his skills.

As time went on, I knew, things may get worse before they got better with the State of California's budget crises, and I really needed to develop a more solid plan for his future. The school's teachers and therapists were only human, and their pink slips were always a constant threat, so they surely didn't want to be the squeaky wheel in demanding or advocating for certain children.

One of Taylor's kindergarten class field trips entailed a variety of car pools all going to a small local theater with a substitute teacher to listen to a holiday concert. I'd been trying to be as active, within reason, as possible in Taylor's activities and trips during the year since the new team was still finding its way, and since I was still looking for a decent paying job, I had the time. So, I volunteered to drive Taylor myself just in case the noise was too much for him and he would want to leave, especially since it was being directed by a substitute teacher that didn't know his sensory issues. I tried to always write to the teacher as first person and cc the rest of the team so at least on my side, everyone was aware of what was going on. I inquired what the team had done to support Taylor as far as prompts were concerned so he was aware that it was a field trip for a concert and that there would be noise. A simple picture story should have been done as a prompt days in advance, showing the car or bus, theater, musical instruments and audience. The picture story was something tangible, visual and sequential so he understood what all was involved in his big field trip and what to expect before he got there. Again, I was always trying to anticipate what could be done to avoid a bad experience for him or any child with sensory issues. As I anticipated, the new team hadn't done any prompting, or given him a simple picture story so he had no idea what he was going to do or what was expected of him. And sure enough, as Taylor and I sat down next to all of his peers in the theater, the music started, and his hands went firmly over his ears. His hands were so tightly held to his head I couldn't remove them. We switched seats to no avail, he was clearly in distress and had no idea what to expect, so as his advocate, I took him out. I held his hand and walked out to the car. "Taylor, baby, I completely respect that you had no idea what you were going to see. No worries. Why don't we go to the park and see if we can find something fun to do there." As he looked at me with his bright blue eyed smile, he knew I understood his world and probably wished his new team did as well.

Our countries ability to compete on a global level for future generations begins with the strong support of our educational system. From early intervention for those that may be at risk to providing the extra support in the classrooms from K-12 for all students. Teachers should be fully accredited and trained to handle teaching all children with or without disabilities before they receive their college diploma. We need to be as proactive as possible for the possibility of the increase of Autism, ADD, ADHD, and other intellectual and developmental disabilities.

Without the internal support systems and funding in all schools throughout the country, I worry we may becoming at risk for more dependence on society by those that needed the support from the beginning. Teachers should have a solid support system in place so they and their students can reach their goals. And their salaries should be commensurate to their training experience, accountability of grades, and time spent in the classroom trying to achieve results. The budget cuts being handed out in California are short term gains on a financial level, but sadly, will have long term consequences especially for those with learning disabilities.

I often think about why we sailed against all odds in a few small ships over a vast sea in the first place. To be united, and create a land full of opportunity for all to be treated equally. My son will go to college if he so chooses, because I will be by his side making sure he has every tool to get there and be as present as any other. He will be in every part of the community that he chooses to be in and I will remain by his side as the proud mother I have grown to become. He will someday make his own choices because we'll make sure he's supported, loved, respected and allowed the opportunity. I want him to feel the way I did fresh out of college. The world is his and his opportunities are endless just as any other child. Given the right supports, education, tools and personal empowerment, Taylor will succeed in anything he so chooses.

CHAPTER 11

Together

What I have learned that my life is a series of snapshots of how Taylor and I cope, how we fit in, and how we attempt to change the world around us for the better. With each new accomplishment Taylor makes, I realize just how far we both have come. It's given me an entirely new framework in life to benefit from and I look forward to the challenges ahead for a change without trepidation. I wouldn't change a day of my life for anything.

Our second Down syndrome group gathering was at Taylor's second Christmas in the Northern countryside of California. It marked another year of raising a child on my own, and I would be lying if I didn't say it was lonely at times, especially around the holidays. I was looking for support and the family feeling we had witnessed two years prior at the Down syndrome Christmas party in San Diego. After four years, the people we met at the gatherings still remain the greatest new family members for which we could ever hope.

The party was at a small community club house in a trailer park with long tables of home-cooked food, several Christmas trees, and children as well as adults with their families. Some individuals had Down syndrome, and some didn't. They were parents, grandparents, aunts, uncles, brothers, sisters and friends alike all arriving with hearts full of hugs and a dish of home-cooked food. It was always a push to scrape up the little money we did have around the holidays, and this year was no different. The financial hardship of bringing something as simple as a couple of pies was difficult for us, but they were our family, and I would sacrifice whatever I had to for the ingredients just the same that I did every day for Taylor. It was about giving and sharing in food, love and support.

Everyone was either laughing and singing or getting to meet Santa Claus for the first time and receiving a gift by the Christmas tree. It was so refreshing to watch everyone talking, sharing and being in a normal atmosphere as friends and families.

One corner of the clubhouse was open for dancing. Another large area had L-shaped buffet tables packed with everything from roast turkey to glazed ham, mashed potatoes and an array of salads, capped at the very end with every home baked cake, pie and cookie assortment imaginable.

Most of us were struggling on a daily basis in one way or another trying to support our families, but this was the one day we all opened our hearts and arms to comfort and appreciate one another. Sacrificing becomes a regular part of your life as a parent. It's just what you do. But on this special day, as we all got together under one big roof, we were just one big happy family. With kids opening their Christmas gifts and Santa adding his "ho ho ho's," parents talked about how their year had been and what they were hoping to accomplish for themselves and for their children in the year ahead. It felt like home to Taylor and I loved watching him dance around and laugh with our friends. Children that played the same as him and had similar features whether they were physical or behavioral. He always seemed at ease and comfortable amongst his Down syndrome group of peers, and so was I.

My whole life before Taylor's birth, I had always been fighting some internal battle with myself. Nothing I ever did was good enough, and I never stopped working myself to the bone. There seemed to be this constant search for something: more money, a bigger house, a better car, or more social status.

And then Taylor came along. With his arrival came the countless parents and children we would meet along our way with much of the same issues we had gone through. As time passed and with each new hurdle we overcame, I learned to soar above them with a greater ease. The love and acceptance within our community followed as well. The more I let go of the label Taylor was given at birth, the clearer our life became and the more it made sense and, the more clarity I had in dealing with those that had never seen a child with Down syndrome. Instead of making things more difficult by being so hard on myself and demanding so much of Taylor, his therapists, and teachers, I learned to embrace them and encourage others to do the same. I know I can't stop every family's struggles completely, but I was beginning to feel this great urge and need to help them through whatever their challenges were because we lived them every day.

Every Christmas party or gathering with our Down syndrome group reminded me of the few times as a little girl when there was peace and calm in my home. I remembered being snowed in, schools closed, and the rolling country hills in a white calm that blanketed our days. The excitement of cooking over our little coal stove in the kitchen when the ice had broken the lines for our electricity and playing Monopoly and Scrabble with my mom and brother. Life was so simple and time seemed to almost stop. I was beginning to crave the peace and tranquility of the simplicities in life, because it was the kind of world Taylor seemed to understand and thrive in. The peace and calm of a simpler life perhaps was better than I ever gave it credit for, and I wanted to know it for Taylor and me going forward.

I still have many of the same worries financially, socially and academically, and time certainly wasn't on our side the way the economy was heading. I was still unemployed, and falling further into debt because of it.

I began cutting the amount of time I was watching mindless television and surfing the computer as well as calling people more instead of texting or e-mailing. Instead of Taylor sitting to watch cartoons or Thomas the Train movies, we sat and played puzzles together or read countless books. Taylor and I read up to eight children's books before his nap or bed every single day, cherishing each one line by line. I'd expanded our hikes and walks outside, turning my Blackberry off and talking to him about all of the things we were seeing, regardless of his lack of ability to respond verbally. He showed me through his eyes and smiles, pointing to each object we found.

Besides learning prioritization, I learned how to set appropriate goals when it came to his outcomes at his school and in our everyday lives. The goals we would set when he first started school were written in his IEP with the expectation of him completing tasks 90-100% of the time over the course of three months. As he progressed and the new team was adjusting, I learned to back off and allow it to read 40-60% of the time. If he reached the 90% success rate, fabulous. If not, we weren't over-setting the expectations for him creating a false sense of success.

I began to dream of reaching out and helping to provide advice, resources and advocacy for all of the parents who were struggling with everything we had endured. If we could help just one family, it would make the last six years of tears vanish. Maybe I could build an inclusion team to travel throughout the United States and help build the foundation for more inclusive schools where the entire community embraced it. Whether it would be through small seminars or a series of workshops, I wanted to help teachers and their students understand the positive attributes children with disabilities had.

After months of searching, I had a 9 AM job interview on the other side of the city for a manager's position within the design industry. It meant cleaning the dust from the shoulders of my suit, rushing Taylor through his breakfast and off to school, and heading into the city in rush hour traffic, all the while angry I was even looking at this job because the salary probably wasn't enough to pay a baby sitter plus the additional costs to get into the city. But, we were almost out of money, and I had to do something. There wasn't a bailout coming and I sure didn't expect to win the lottery.

As I ran through the school yard in my high heels and suit with Taylor in my arms, I felt overwhelmingly saddened I would have to employ someone to do this instead of me. It felt like I was selling myself out to sell and push products I didn't even like rather than helping children like Taylor. I entered the classroom door to find all of Taylor's peers cheering because he just walked in and narrowly missed the late bell. I wanted to experience more of these kinds of cheers with him, not away from him.

The road into the city was longer than I remembered this time. There were more cars and everyone seemed to be in a giant hurried frenzy. My chest was slightly pressed and my breath seemed a bit short. The stress of the commute was apparent. I made it at three minutes to 9:00 and was able to regain my composure before I entered the interview.

There was something so bittersweet about the showroom. The former owner was the mentor to the owner of the firm I was let go from the previous Christmas. Although I personally had no desire whatsoever to take the job, two and half hours later, I had an offer to not only manage the showroom, but with a preference to work in their corporate office. The salary would have to be revisited, because as I suspected, it wasn't enough to cover the increase in commuting expenditures and Taylor's care.

We shook hands and agreed to revisit the salary within the week. I said my goodbyes to the staff I had just met and a gave cordial thank you to the corporate head that allowed me her time. As I sank into the seat of my car in front of the showroom, I knew. I knew I would rather cut off my right arm than take another job where I was at the mercy of corporate heads. Those who would think nothing of tossing a single mother and her child to the curb at the stroke of a pen. The world of luxury design was no longer mine, and if I was to be true to myself, I couldn't do this to Taylor.

I had no idea how I could support both of us financially by my "philosophy" of inclusion; all I knew was I couldn't go back to where I had been. After twenty-three years of working to be elite in the design world and a portion of society, I was now prouder to say I was turning my back on it and them. I was more proud to be a mother of a beautiful little boy who had a disability. Or was it really an ability—an ability the majority of society doesn't understand. My son seemed to have an extraordinary ability to teach the most important attribute: compassion.

The ride home was sunny and warm. The drive across the bridge gave me enormous pangs of relief. I was going home . . . . home to my new path and journey against financial odds because it was the right thing to do for my son and all children and families that may need me. I was trained in my early design years to do the design first and the money would follow. And so, I would embrace the same philosophy in our pursuit of inclusion.

Taylor blasted through his classroom door as he did every day when I picked him up, jumping into my arms for a huge hug and then running to the nearest drain to throw something in it. All he cared about was seeing me at the end of the day and a regular routine. So, as I patiently guided him towards the parking lot, he grabbed as many tiny stones as possible, tapping on six poles bordering the school driveway. Every day the same tap on the same six poles. Then I would pick him up from behind so he could reach over the tall steel mesh fence to throw another rock into the small canal abutting the parking lot. As he's tapping on the poles, I saw our friend Caroline being lifted from her wheel chair by her mother, Briana, as she walked to their car. Her chin was resting on Briana's shoulder when her eyes locked onto mine. It was like she knew my inner turmoil, fears and hopes. Her stare seemed to say, "I know." I smiled back and knew. This was just the beginning of a beautiful life with her, my son, and so many other children that needed a voice. That is the day I really knew what the rest of my life looked like. And I never turned back.

CHAPTER 12

Vermont

My mind began to flash back over the past seven years with images of constant struggles rather than images of happiness and fun. One of my clearest memories was lying in the safety of my hot bubble bath the night before Taylor was born. The door was locked, my head under water to drown out my husband's yelling, and I was talking to Taylor in my belly. The steam rose from the faucet and the heat of the water blanketed us in complete calm. I imagined his little toes, legs, arms, and his little champagne grape-sized fingers. I wanted to make sure I was connected to every part of his body, reassuring myself he would be a healthy little baby boy. And then when I reached his head, his mind, it was absolutely clear to me something was wrong. I remember every last detail of this moment as I gently rubbed my belly. *Taylor baby, something is going on here, but, wow, you sure are going to be a really fun kid, aren't you?!* It was almost as if both of us were laughing simultaneously. I knew something was different about my child, and yet it only gave me strength because I knew how much he would need me. He knew more than I, his laughter and smile would forever be our strength and bond.

More snapshots appeared, flashing like light bulbs in my mind as I started to think of our move out of California. I flashed to the courtroom when my ex-husband was being led away in shackles by a bailiff after the verdict of thirteen jurors was reached. He was convicted of three counts of domestic violence against me while I was eight and nine months pregnant. I then flashed to my hotel room the night the verdict was reached. I stood over my beautiful sleeping baby crying into a washcloth because the

121

tissues were too frail for my tears, thinking of the monster I had married, feeling the pains of guilt for my son, who may grow up without a father.

Flashes of all the years of meetings at Taylor's school pleading for someone to just do their job and help my son access the simplest things in his classroom. Another snapshot was pushing his little stroller past our beautiful neighborhood restaurants with the smells of garlic, steaks and fresh baked bread. Knowing that we wouldn't be able to afford to sit down amongst the crowd and taste the beauty of someone else's cooking and fine food.

My final snapshot was the little girl we had seen at our local public swimming pool. She was about five feet away from Taylor pointing at him, jumping up and down laughing. She was laughing and pointing saying, "You're funny looking! Look how funny that boy looks!" I held onto Taylor as tight as I could, trying to find the mother of the little girl to confront her about her child's horrific behavior. I was in complete shock crying for my son that was too young to know the pain.

My child saved my life from everything that was wrong with it. He became the facilitator all along, not my adversity. I was just finally seeing what he had been showing me all of these years. He showed me the kindness of life and the safety that lived within it. I had to know true pain before I knew what real love was.

And so, the process of building an inclusive life for Taylor began one Thursday afternoon after seeing the gaze in little Caroline's eyes. I needed to help her mom so we didn't have to sit across from each other, crying over how exhausted we were caring for our children. It wasn't our children that were the exhaustion; it was the system and lack of help for our children and us as parents.

Our condo went on the market the next day and I began to sell anything that I could to put towards moving costs. From all of my years of research, New Hampshire and Vermont were doing the most cutting edge educational programs for inclusion within the United States. I applied to the University of Vermont for my Master's Degree in Early Childhood Special Education and sent them some recent writings along with my application. I had no idea what I was doing at the time, only I had to be the change in my son's life.

Every single day Taylor was at school, I tirelessly searched Craigslist for places to live, and Googled hundreds of towns in Vermont and New Hampshire to see where the best inclusive schools were and what community seemed fitting for both of us. I spoke to families, advocates and educators throughout the United States and everything kept leading me back to Vermont as the best overall in community acceptance and support of people with disabilities.

The University of Vermont accepted my application June 2nd, 2011. My home sold four weeks later. I had begun telling Taylor what our new life was going to look like and how much fun we were going to have. I showed him the beautiful rolling hills of Vermont dotted with cows and giant red barns. We talked about a new school and how many great friends he was going to have and all of the great things they would do together.

As our plans were starting to fall into place, the director of the Early Childhood Program at The University of Vermont called and said they had one final opening for a scholarship for their Master's Degree Program in Early Childhood Special Education. Professor Jenkins changed the course of Taylor's and my life forever that day. It was only for in-state tuition and I had no idea how I would subsidize the out-of-state cost difference but, I felt it was the greatest possibility yet for a new life. I tearfully and gratefully accepted without hesitation. I could finally study the inner workings of education, and especially in helping educate myself about a world I felt I knew so little about. I was curious if my philosophy of inclusion was in fact crazy or if it really could be done easily if everyone were just on the same page.

Best of all, in my preliminary research, I had found the most perfect elementary school about six miles from the University with one of the best Special Education programs in the area. Most of the students from the University were P.C.A.'s (personal care assistants) who used their free time to care for children like my son Taylor to earn credits for their own various educational programs. They were students studying to be physical therapists, occupational therapists, speech therapists, as well as teachers. The most exciting part: not only were they able to watch Taylor while I worked and studied, but they would also be working with him in his new elementary school as aides a.k.a. para-educators. His elementary school's proximity to the University allowed everyone to work together in every capacity of a real community just like the one I dreamed of for so many years.

As Professor Jenkins described every component of support I would receive as a single parent of a child with a disability, I swore I was dreaming and the tears flowed even more. Someone believed in my son and me and was giving us a chance to start a fresh new life away from all of the pains of the past seven years. Taylor would finally have equal opportunities and support.

July 21, 2011, I had finally finished packing the moving truck, taking the bare essentials of toys and clothing in the car for the three thousand mile drive to Vermont. The sense of relief was just beginning to surface, yet I knew the warrior mom in me couldn't let my guard down until we had actually stepped into our new home. Taylor wasn't quite sure what was going on, but I made sure to keep his cherished toys and Thomas the Tank Engine trains and track visible in the car as a sense of comfort and familiarity.

The cooler was packed with four cases of his favorite vanilla yogurt, apple juice, almond milk, oatmeal, spaghetti and Pediasure. I had found a fantastic little skillet that I could bring into our hotel room every night and make his spaghetti as well as his morning oatmeal, keeping some sense of normalcy in his new six day "routine" in driving East.

Our last night in our little town was at a sweet little hotel with a swimming pool just below the beautiful local mountain separating us from the ocean. One of my dearest friends, Fiona, mother of Brian, Brady and Gunner met us at the hotel for one last play date for the kids, and one last get together for she and I. Gunner had been the wonderful boy we had observed when I was thinking of placing Taylor into a general education classroom, and he and Taylor had become fast friends. I would miss all of them dearly, but I also knew how much Fiona struggled like I did trying to find a smooth path in our little elementary school. I could help her more once I began my studies and connected with people within the field of education on the University level. It just affirmed I had made the right decision as we said our tearful good byes, and I promised to study as hard as I could to be able to help her from the other side. I began to think of how much of a warrior Fiona and I had to be, for Gunner and Taylor.

The next morning, I settled Taylor into the back seat of our little car with his two musical popping ball machine toys and a talking Elmo doll. As I closed his car door, and walked around to the driver's seat, I looked at the bright blue California sky, smelling the misty air of redwoods and eucalyptus trees, and said goodbye to a geography I had fallen so in love with. Every facet of California's coastline was breathtaking and I was going to miss it. And then, I looked back at Taylor as I sat down in my driver's seat and knew this was just the beginning of our life together, not an end by any means.

The journey from state to state was nothing short of hilarious. Every night, after driving eight intense hours without anyone to turn the wheel over to, I would bring in our suitcase, his toilet seat, the cooler of his food, skillet, my computer, handbag, toys and a case of wine my best friend gave me as a going away present. All the while, trying to flag Taylor as he ran to check things out every time we got out of the car. I'm not sure what was funnier, carrying all of our stuff into the room night after night, or the never ending sounds from his toys for eight hours straight in the car including flying plastic balls from his ball popping machines. It kept him entertained and happy, and just one more sacrifice as a parent! We laughed at the silliest things state after state as he remained a trooper never fussing or whining, but seemingly liking our newest adventure.

Night after night, we rolled into a different hotel with a pool so he could swim and get his energy out from sitting in a cramped car all day. Our amazing Florida family had given us the money to make the drive, so we were actually able to stay in some really nice Marriott Hotels and Best Westerns, with a decent hot meal for me at the end of each day.

It felt like the dynamic of Thelma and Louise with each new state line we crossed, getting closer and closer to a new life without fear, without fighting, and with only endless possibilities. I finally felt free and it showed in Taylor's behavior and happiness. We were making as much of a daily routine as possible in our six day drive, and he was actually eating and playing as he would have at home, because we kept it structured stopping and starting at the same time every day, and swimming every night.

As we drove through the hundreds of miles of endless cornfields in Nebraska, I looked into the rearview mirror that was always pointed down so I could see Taylor. I had a tiny wave of panic overwhelm me as I said, "Oh my gosh baby, I think you're momma is crazy! What have I done? I've sold our home with no real income to support us, and we're moving 3200 miles across the country to live in a place that we have never even been to! And the worst part is, these cornfields feel like they are never going to end!" The next thing I knew we were both laughing our heads off. It was his skill and he was really good at it. Through thick and thin, Taylor always laughed at his ridiculously stressed out mom and kept it real. He knows everything I am saying and has an innate ability to always put my mind and heart at rest, regardless of his lack of words.

Six days and 3200 miles later, we were loading our car onto a small ferry barge from upstate New York over Lake Champlain, to a small town in the lush countryside of Vermont. The people were incredibly friendly to Taylor, allowing him to peer over the edge of the barge as its waves crashed against the pontoon edges. The boat's American flag was flapping in the wind against a bright clear blue July afternoon. Feelings of freedom, relief, happiness and hope were absolutely overwhelming as we approached the Vermont shoreline. Taylor and I were finally free to live our lives with people that would accept us and help us. We stepped back into the car and slowly drove off the barge once it had docked, and I saw the beautiful sign I had been waiting for, "Welcome to Vermont!" I said, "Yeah! We did it Taylor! We made it to Vermont, our new home!" The tears welled in my eyes as I sighed a giant sigh of relief.

As we settled into our townhouse, it was absolutely perfect for Taylor and me. It was six miles from the University and one mile from his wonderful elementary school. Our small neighborhood had a safe and friendly community feel to it with a wonderful swimming pool for Taylor during the summers. Our plowing and shoveling was all done through the association, so that was one less worry I had to deal with during the harsh long winters I had been warned of.

I took Taylor to tour the outside of his new school and playground so he was familiar with it, as well as all of the other local playgrounds and stores. Getting him as familiar as possible with his new environment became our full-time job, as well as building his new routine. We went to play on the grounds at my University as well just so he was familiar with mommy's new surroundings too. This was about us, not just me.

I instantly noticed one of the greatest qualities of Vermonters was how kind and accepting everyone was. As we walked into the post office to get our mail every day, people actually ran to be able to open the door for us. At our local Wal-Mart one Saturday, I was having a hard time fitting something into my car when a mother with three children ran to ask if she could help me. Everywhere we went, people were no longer staring at Taylor, but saying hello and being sure to always be respectful of their words in talking to him or me. This was a community that embraced everyone not for social status or something in return, but rather to be a kind human being. We were no longer singled out in a crowd, but a part of the crowd.

Every morning I dropped Taylor off at school, I walked him inside so I could talk to his Special Education Director as well as his aide to catch up on how things were going. Every afternoon, Taylor and his new found friends rode the bus which would drop him off ten feet from our front door. He was no longer running out of the classroom or hiding under desks the way he did in his last school, but rather sitting amongst his peers and working side by side with them.

He was given the same multi-level curriculum as all the other children in his classroom, only this time it was modified with a variety of accommodations and supports. He worked on the same content as the other children, just with different outcomes according to his developmental ability. Taylor was thrilled and embracing almost every piece of his new education because they were giving him educational challenges. Within four months, he was adding and subtracting. He was excelling in math, music and art, as well as learning the basic skills in gym class like kicking the soccer ball, climbing the playground's ladders, and throwing and catching the ball. Instead of putting Taylor into a box because he had a disability, every single teacher and therapist worked on the skills they wanted to see him accomplish. And it worked!

For the first time in Taylor's education, I looked forward to his IEP team meetings because they accepted me as the parent expert. I was the expert of my son because day in and day out I was around him more than anyone else. Our IEP meetings weren't about anyone being right or wrong, but more of a collaboration between all of us about what we thought, what we could do better, or what support I needed at home for Taylor.

Taylor's new team consisted of an Occupational Therapist, Physical Therapist, Speech and Language Therapist, Special Education Director, Aide and of course, his General Education Teacher. The biggest difference with everyone including his General Education Teacher was that they all had been raised since their early childhood in inclusive settings, and they also were fully trained in Special Education on several different levels. We weren't necessarily starting over again with Taylor even though he was a new student in a new school with a whole new team because they already had enough experience with children like Taylor.

Taylor's IEP Special Education services for his second year of Kindergarten were forty-five minutes per week for Speech & Language Therapy, forty-five minutes per week for Occupational Therapy, forty-five per week for one on one with the Special Education Teacher and a full time aide. His new IEP for first grade included one hundred and eighty minutes per week for one-to-one instruction with his Special Education Teacher, forty-five minutes per week for the Special Education Teacher's personal case management time, sixty minutes per week for Speech & Language Therapy, thirty minutes per week for Occupational Therapy, thirty minutes per week for Physical Therapy, plus a full time aide, and of course the additional support of his well-trained, General Education Teacher across all school settings. Besides the one-to-one therapy sessions, the therapists were also embedding Taylor's goals and objectives in every facet of his program with his peers. The classroom size is only sixteen children with one teacher and one aide in Taylor's class in Vermont, compared to twenty-six children with one teacher and one aide in his previous classroom in California. The difference between the two was incredible and so was the amount of progress Taylor was making in his new school.

The primary support used in Taylor's school is PBIS (Positive Behavioral Interventions & Supports) which is a school-wide approach to creating a positive and safe climate in which students can learn and grow. It's used throughout the entire school environment, as well as the lunchroom and playground. The overall concept is creating a positive approach when addressing the discipline of all children. The administration, teachers, therapists and counselors all work in collaboration to teach and support the behavioral expectations at school. It's based on Three Tiers. The first, Tier One: "The Universal" level, is designed to support all students. The second, Tier Two is designed for approximately 15% of students who will need a more "targeted" level of support through small-group interventions. And the last level, Tier Three includes about 5%, of children who may require support at "intensive" level, which involves individualized and specialized interventions.

Taylor's last school and many others throughout the country were beginning the interventions of discipline at the Third Tier when it was crises intervention time. In other words, instead of pre-teaching the bottom tiers and pre-teaching the expected behaviors at school and with the parents at home, they were only treating the problem after the antecedent spurred disciplinary action. The model is basically a pyramid of One Tier at the bottom filled with pre-teaching, the second then becomes a slight intervention if the teaching wasn't enough, and the third was a bit of "crisis" mode if the teaching and discipline wasn't getting through to the behavior. The model is an evidenced-based approach and as I witnessed firsthand with Taylor, an extraordinary approach for all children, especially those with special needs. It was the same approach we had adopted at home, with an expectation of behavior. By pre-teaching him, it allowed him the time he needed to process what he may or may not be doing wrong.

The other most exciting, and "state of the art" educational adoption in the State of Vermont, is the *Common Core State Standard Initiative* for grades K-12. Per the Vermont public Education website, the description is as follows:

> "No Child Left Behind brought accountability—but not necessarily consistency—in the adoption of standards across state lines. As Americans have become more mobile, our children face increasing difficulty in moving from state to state or school to school, finding varying standards and related curriculum in the core areas of mathematics and language arts. The Common Core Standards Initiative is the beginning of a national effort to ameliorate those differences. Focused in the areas of mathematics, reading, writing, speaking and listening, the Common Core Standards are internationally benchmarked and designed to better

prepare our young people for 21st century college and
career opportunities."

For years, I had been led to believe the State of California
was as state of the art in education as it got, and it was the main
reason why I worked so hard to stay there for Taylor. Only in
coming to Vermont did I truly understand where many of our
incredible educational programs were actually coming from. It is
a place that doesn't care so much about who is right or wrong,
but what is right for the common good of the people.

CHAPTER 13

Closure

Though it feels like yesterday, I remember driving across country a little over ten years ago from my Florida home of thirteen years to Lake Tahoe, California with my little, black, curly-haired cocker spaniel Rufus leading the way as my furry co-pilot and best friend. After the tragedy of 9/11 and the loss of my interior design company after the initial economic fallout, I was ready to start a new life away from my sixteen hour, seven days a week company and start fresh in a more serene environment. I was filled with hopes and dreams of meeting my future husband, settling down and beginning a family of my own in one of my favorite places in the world.

My memories of Lake Tahoe as a little girl on holiday were filled with families hiking, biking, water skiing and having the time of their lives in the awe-inspiring high altitude mountains surrounding the lake. When I grew up, I planned to meet Mr. Perfect who was athletic, intelligent, kind, and shared the same passion for living life as I did. We would have our two children, a Labrador, and live happily ever after behind our perfect little white picket fence.

Now, as I reflect back over the past seven and a half years with Taylor, I realize the sunny, perfect images I once held so clear in my mind, of what my life was "supposed" to look like, are now completely different images. They are still filled with bright, sunny, fun days, but the landscape is different. My values were different then, as were my wants and needs because I was now a parent. My son has given me a gift of love and compassion that I never could have imagined. Surely not in my drive West ten years ago, would I ever have thought how fulfilled my life would be thanks to the presence of a very special little boy. Our journey together has been long and challenging at times, but worth every minute because we did it together.

As I think of what I foresee in the long term for Taylor and myself, my visions and hopes are clear because of all of our experiences leading up to this point in our lives. I have no regrets, and I will always hold California very dear and close to my heart. It just was not in the best interest for my son to grow up in our suburban Northern California town. It wasn't only his educational issues that concerned me, but more the community's lack of acceptance. As much as it pained me to leave California, the pain of staying was even greater in the best interest of my son. His exclusion from the community far outweighed a beautiful geography, great restaurants and fabulous weather. In everything I had learned in California and about myself, I had developed one very distinct phobia: I couldn't handle anyone not accepting and helping my son. The thought created an anxiety within me both impossible to comprehend and impossible to accept with the little resources I had. I was in constant worry of him being teased or not included in his classroom as well as the rest of his general education setting. I just couldn't fathom how a system and a community could make things so difficult for a mother that was just trying to do right by her child.

With the birth of my son, and the struggles we had endured along the way, I realized we needed a locale filled with advanced schools and diverse communities. We needed a state that valued education, community relationships, and doing what was right for the greater good of all people, regardless of their own self interests.

We were now completely surrounded with true inclusion in the state of Vermont. I have to laugh because after all of the years of studying inclusion and fighting for it, it's such a common practice in Vermont that the word is rarely used. We don't have to really talk about it because it is so deeply embedded in the community.

As Taylor settled into his school, I did as well in my new Special Education studies at the University of Vermont. In many ways, sitting through the lectures with some of the greatest minds in education, I felt it was almost a review of what I a had already been experiencing. After seven and a half years of advocating for Taylor and living with him, fighting for him, I had already earned my master's degree. Now, my knowledge and studies at the university level just had a grade behind it and diploma at the end.

To supplement our income, I began working with a dear friend and former business acquaintance named Stephan as a U.S. representative for four different textile mills in Italy. It allowed me to work from home, finish my master's degree and, most importantly, be home for Taylor when he got off his school bus every day. The income wasn't much, but every day I built more and more accounts, knowing there would be a reward if I worked hard and stuck with it. I just wanted Taylor to be in a happy, loving and stable home with the full support of his incredible school and amazing local hospitals, physicians and therapists. I also took a full twelve credit course load at the university, worked in the Dean of Education's office for work study to be able to buy groceries and all the while balancing my textile business and meeting Taylor's every day needs.

The state of California had picked up the burden of Taylor's initial hospital bills from his birth which was well over $86,000, plus his Medicaid coverage for seven years but our financial struggles had been ongoing. I was facing bankruptcy, living paycheck to paycheck, and struggling to keep food on the table, at times forced to go on welfare when even that became impossible. Yet the man who had helped create Taylor wasn't paying child support and never had; the state system never went after him for reimbursement. At the time of our divorce in 2006, he was making over $130,000. Had he provided child support, I never would have had to turn to welfare or fear how I would continue to provide for Taylor. My fear of the domestic violence and potential harm to Taylor lived with me for seven years, never allowing me the courage to file for child support.

In October of 2011, I finally filed for child support for I could no longer allow him to control me, and I had to let go of my fears for Taylor's sake. With thousands of miles between us, I gained the sense of safety necessary to address Taylor's father's negligence. To protect our location, we red flagged every piece of paper that was sent with Taylor and I's contact information and address. The case was transferred from my prior county courts in suburbia to the courts of the Northern California wine country region where my ex-husband was now residing.

I had sold our condo in California months prior which paid for our trip across country, some outstanding bills and the first few months of living expenses in Vermont. The last of our money went to babysitters so I could go to my night classes while Taylor stayed home. My stress level was almost non-existent, and I was able to accomplish everything with greater ease because my son was safe, happy and in the best school system I could find. As the months went by and Thanksgiving approached, we didn't have a dime for food, and I had just fallen two weeks behind in rent.

My father and step mother hadn't seen Taylor in about three years, but surprised us by making the long drive for Thanksgiving. It was a wonderful visit, filled with warmth and happiness. As my father said good-bye, he handed me $500.00 in cash and said they would pay our rent until I finished my graduate program. The tears rose in my eyes. Finally, my family was understanding the magnitude of how difficult our everyday lives were and how hard I had worked trying to provide everything that my son needed.

Christmas soon followed, only this year, it was different than any other. We didn't have much, but with the falling of the beautiful fluffy white snow, and the ambiance of a Norman Rockwell painting on every street and in every neighborhood, we were finally both at peace. Every night, just after dark, we drove around the neighborhoods with Taylor in his pajamas and bulky winter coat to look at the incredible Christmas lights. Every single house in every neighborhood was completely trimmed and Taylor was ecstatic with so much visual stimulation!

The months went by with still no word from child support. The Vermont child support office said California was a bit slow in responding, and so the dance began. Phone call after phone call, e-mail after e-mail it—was always a different story. Finally, on March 8, 2012, I received notification of a hearing from the Northern California County Court for child support. I needed to call a number in Los Angeles to set up a court call, so I could have a live feed to the court room in California while I was in the child support office in Vermont. I couldn't afford a lawyer, so I would have to represent myself.

Prior to the first hearing, the case manager of child support services in California called to inform me that my ex-husband was fighting his obligation to pay child support. Of course, I thought; one of the many reasons I hadn't tried seven years ago. I was still in constant fear of the man, and after he signed away visitation in order to not pay child support after Taylor was born, I knew this case could possibly be a waste of time. He would do anything to avoid paying, including moving his money around so it wasn't traceable. The case manager proceeded to state that his child support payment calculated to $1345.00 per month since he had no visitation. His tax returns had numerous "suspect" deductions which I could only imagine, if challenged, would show an even greater obligation to pay child support. She gently explained that since my ex-husband was claiming he was a sub-contractor, they were having a hard time verifying his real income.

Even as my anxiety grew, so did my determination. On Taylor's behalf I was asking for child support to cover child care expenses, (above what Medicaid covered for a child with a disability for personal care costs), health insurance so Taylor wouldn't have to still be on a state funded health insurance program, as well as $6000.00 for the cost of a service dog that Taylor was accepted for and needed. I explained all of Taylor's special needs and answered what few questions the case manager had.

Our first over the phone hearing was May 6th. The judge was brief as he reviewed our paperwork and proceeded to ask my ex-husband how he was supporting himself given a declared income of $545.00 and living expenses of $3200.00 per month. My ex-husband stated he had been living off of his mother's inheritance, and was having a very difficult time with income from his sub-contracted job. The judge began to dig a little deeper asking if he was current on his mortgage, credit cards, and any other bills. My ex-husband stated, yes, he was in fact current on his mortgage, bills, and that he had no credit card debt.

As I sat on the other end of the telephone line, I was shaking and seething at the same time, thinking of this man, my ex-husband, last seen with shackles around his ankles and handcuffs on his wrists being led out of the courtroom after his domestic violence conviction. The image still burned in my mind as I heard his voice for the first time since that dark day. And now, I had to listen to this heartless man lie and fight not to pay for food, clothing and shelter for his beautiful son. After all of Taylor's surgeries, our debt from attorney's bills and medical bills, it was beyond sickening. By the end of the call, we had nothing resolved, other than the judge requesting me to furnish the exact amount and receipts for the child care expenses I paid above and beyond what Medicaid paid.

The second court call on May 10th was just as brief as the first, as the judge reviewed my expenses of $433.00 per month for child care that I paid out of my pocket so I could attend my graduate night classes. Next, he reviewed my ex-husband's Income and Expense statement once again and decided since my ex-husband couldn't verify his income, the judge would base the child support obligation on a minimum wage job. As the judge said, "Mr. Smith, I suggest if your sub-contractor job isn't providing you with any income, you get a paying salaried job immediately. We will base your child support amount on the new job at a minimum wage rate." As the judge turned his attention back to me, he asked if I had anything further to say. And so, I requested the availability of private health insurance from my ex-husband's insurance policy for Taylor as well as half of the service dog expense. The judge's response was just as brief and dismissive as it was the first time when I requested it in the prior hearing. He wanted documentation of the medical necessity of a service dog for Taylor to warrant such an extraordinary expense. Clearly this man had absolutely no idea of the cost to raise a child with special needs, how much extra time and care a child like Taylor required, nor any apparent prior experience with a case involving a child with special needs. He wanted more documentation from me, rather than the man who was hiding his income. And so, another court date was set for May 25th.

For May 25th, I had the prescription from Taylor's pediatrician for Taylor's service dog with Taylor's diagnosis and a copy of the service dog contract. Upon review of the doctor's prescription, I had blacked out the pediatrician's address as well as last name as I was allowed to do to protect our exact location due to the domestic violence. The judge demanded to know the pediatrician's name and address in an open forum rather than in his private chambers, thereby endangering our safety and the California court order. I clearly stated I didn't want to disclose the information due to my ex-husband's prior domestic violence conviction, and I reminded him I had a Family Violence Indicator activated on my case. Therefore, it was previously court ordered I didn't have to disclose any personal addresses, names, etc. pertaining to my case on any paperwork to ensure my child's safety as well as my own. For whatever reason, he wouldn't back down and he denied the validity of the pediatrician's prescription, stating that it wasn't enough information to warrant such a high expense. He also negated the other substantiation of the contract from the service dog provider detailing the need for a service dog for Taylor's neurological condition including the section where it referred to the actual article of research based evidence. I even brought up compliance with I.D.E.A. (Individuals with Disabilities Education Act) for Taylor to have a service dog to better access his education, and ADA (American Disabilities Act) which clearly defines the justification for a person with a neurological disability to attain a service dog. Still the judge refused and, once again, the court hearing was rescheduled so I could provide further evidence that my son needed a service dog. He also ordered my ex-husband to bring evidence of availability of private health insurance for Taylor through his employer.

Under duress, I disclosed the name and address of Taylor's pediatrician, jeopardizing Taylor and I's safety. After years of protecting my child from potential harm from my ex-husband, a judge in five minutes or less compromised everything. I never should have filed for support for Taylor and I was beginning to feel like a fool for even trying. It was just one more fight I didn't have the time or energy for, and worst of all, without a private attorney, I was failing in getting the proper amount of $1345.00 per month that they originally told me Taylor was eligible for. How many other single mothers had to fight this hard just to get the basic needs for their children met? How many other parents had to fight for every little morsel of help? I just couldn't understand how a judicial system could be so broken

After eight months of paperwork, I finally received the final court order for child support on June 5, 2012. Based on the minimum wage my ex-husband had been told to find, according to the judge, the monthly child support came to $251.00 and the child care expense to be paid was $217.00 totaling $468.00 per month. That wouldn't even cover Taylor's special food items for a month. Once again, I was caught in a broken system. I had no money for a private attorney to represent Taylor, and my sleepless nights of anxiety were beginning once again.

Shortly after I received the court order of support, the Northern California County child support office called to say they had a request from my ex-husband. He wondered if I would agree to not have a court order for child support, garnishing his earnings. Instead, he would just send Taylor's payments every month to me directly. As I processed this ridiculous request, furious and frustrated, I quickly figured it out: he was running scared. If his earnings were garnished, child support services would see how much income he was really making in his sub-contracted job, rather than what he was "telling" them he was making.

At the end of the day, the most important person is my son, Taylor and in times like these, I needed to remind myself of this and remain calm about the situation to my ex-husband. I would no longer allow my emotions of fear and anxieties to overpower me, but rather empower me to do the right thing for my son. I have been his sole provider for almost eight years and sold almost everything we had, including our home so I could provide the best life possible for him with the best resources for his special needs. If I had it to do all over again, I wouldn't change a moment of our experiences because it has made us who we are today. My focus needs to remain changing the things I am able to change for the greater good and letting go of the things that I cannot. I cannot change how my ex-husband feels about a child he conceived who may not fit his image of what a son should be. And I most certainly could not change the fact that he would forever fight sending child support. As I pick my battles as any other warrior mom, I know battling my ex-husband in any way for my son is not one I choose to fight anymore. After everything I had been through, fighting the various government and state systems as well as a dead beat dad, I deserved closure and wanted to move on with my life with the one person that mattered, Taylor.

June 21, 2012 we had yet another court hearing to establish the necessity for the service dog as well as coverage of private health insurance by my ex-husband. The judge as usual, began with me. I had previously faxed a letter from the pediatrician stating the following:

To Whom it May Concern,

Please accept my request for a service dog for Taylor. Taylor is a wonderful seven-year-old child with Down syndrome and Autism. He has a very supportive mother, and a supportive elementary school. As a part of his Autism, Taylor has a lot of difficulty making emotional connections with others. When he visits me, he spends the whole time playing around the room in his own world, but does not make eye contact with me, and he does not interact with others. He is emotionally connected with his mother. He has a number of challenges in his life from medical conditions. However, the one that will likely post the greatest challenge for him will be his difficulty with interpersonal relationships. Without the ability to interact well with others, he will have a much greater difficulty in his life getting medical care, advocating for himself, and forming meaningful relationships. I believe that a service dog would be one of the best ways for him to work on making emotional connections. This small, albeit nontraditional medical intervention could work wonders for him. Thank you for your consideration. Please let me know if you have any further questions.

Dr. M.

After reviewing the letter, the judge asked my ex-husband if he had seen it, to which my ex-husband replied no. As the judge was about to hand over the letter, I reminded him it was to be a redacted version, without the pediatrician's name and address per our non-disclosure order. The judge quickly deemed this unnecessary as the pediatrician was not a part of the non-disclosure, only my son and I. My argument was that our town in Vermont was very small and any disclosed information of our whereabouts might jeopardize the safety of my son and I. "Well, this is a large geography, and I hardly think disclosing the name and town of the pediatrician warrants merit to redacting the letter," he replied. "What you are also saying is that the pediatrician is in harms way." The anger within me began to boil as the warrior mother began to emerge. "Your honor, with all due respect to the court, if anything happens to my son because the court disclosed our personal information, I will hold the State

141

of California as well as this court responsible." I was not going to be bullied by anyone anymore, let alone a judge. I had had enough. Of course, he wasn't thrilled that I "threatened him" per his words, however the pediatrician's letter was redacted and handed to my ex-husband. No one would push me around when it came to my child; the court room and everyone else within its walls needed to know that.

After careful review, the judge referred to the last statement of the letter: "This small, albeit nontraditional medical intervention could work wonders for him." He did not think this last statement substantiated the evidence to prove the need for a service dog. Therefore, he requested another round of paperwork from me. This time, I was to provide empirical evidence—based research papers from medical journals to further justify that a child with Autism would benefit from a service dog. Perhaps if I weren't reading peer-reviewed evidence-based research papers every single day for my master's degree, I would have shuddered at the thought of what that meant. However, his honor was talking to the queen of research, and I now found this quite a wonderful game of cat and mouse. Not only would I provide one, I would send him every single article and research-based paper I could find. I was quite sure in the end it would still be denied, however perhaps it would empower me or someone else to go to the council of ADA so this never happened again to any parent with a child with a neurological disorder requiring a service dog.

As we then moved back to my ex-husband and his court order to provide private health insurance for Taylor, it became brief. My ex-husband said because Taylor was out of state, he was unable to provide private health insurance for him. His employer did not offer health insurance, and he therefore had his own insurance. Once again, the judge did not balk, but rather dismissed the request and adjourned the hearing. In his closing he repeated his request for me to send the research based articles to him and said he may court order the allowance for my ex-husband to call my son's pediatrician after the articles were read to confirm the necessity of the service dog which would negate the previous non-disclosure court order protecting my son's and my whereabouts and further jeopardizing our safety. None of it was making sense, and probably never would. I was exhausted and tired of fighting systems that weren't designed for people that were actually doing the right thing by their children. It wasn't worth another battle or fight distracting me from what I am better at: advocating for those that need me. I was ready to move on with my life and leave this mess behind. I at least won the $468.00 per month support for Taylor even though it should have been more. And the craziest part was Taylor would continue to have to use government and state funds for his health insurance, while his paternal father escaped yet another loophole in the system by not being court ordered to provide private health insurance for him. If I had a private attorney representing Taylor, I am sure the end results would have been dramatically different.

Walking out of the local Vermont child support office, I felt like a huge monkey had finally hopped off my back and I was ready to take on the next chapter of our lives. It was a relief to know I advocated the best I could for my son and I made some progress in doing so. This was my new life with him and a much better direction for my life's work and dedication. Vermont was a place where the past of my own prior life could hold no memory and we could finally be free.

I am Taylor's mother and with that has come great responsibility, just like any parent. I laugh at my own quote; "I just don't want to mess up my son's life."

My dear friend, Charlie recently heard me say it and laughed. "Kim," he said "no parent intentionally or unintentionally wants to mess up their kid's life. That's a tall order. Stop being so hard on yourself. You do the best you can and pray."

In my mind, no matter what I do, it will never be good enough. I love my son so deeply and am so passionate for those like him; it's almost a nagging pain in my heart. But, because of this passion, I have grown in ways I never thought possible for myself. I have learned to accept everyone for who they are, without labels. I may not always agree with their point of view, or opinions, but I have learned to value people just as they are without judgment.

Life for me is a series of snapshots of experiences. My experiences and the lessons I have learned while living them are what I remember now. I've learned to filter out the challenges and difficult times. Embracing rather the memory and experience of how I lived after the tough times had passed. I'm learning to be in the present moment as a parent and enjoy the little things. I laugh more at our obstacles, because Taylor has taught me more than anyone that you just can't sweat the small stuff. The most important aspects in anyone's life are health, wellness, friends and family. For this you simply cannot buy, nor can you ever replace. At least that's what my son taught me, and I so agree.

Every moment I have spent with Taylor is an amazing journey. Even through the challenges of his surgeries, medical appointments, therapies, and schooling issues, I have learned things beyond my comprehension in a very short amount of time. We have grown together in forming a great mother and son bond that in itself has been an incredible experience. With each experience comes gratefulness. I am genuinely grateful for every memory because it has taught me a whole world I never knew existed. It is a world of people who wear their hearts on their sleeves and who hold a genuine passion for happiness and compassion. My experience with Down syndrome has nothing to do with being down. It's a world of people filled with hugs and love. My son and all of his friends like him have so much to teach us about compassion, honesty and a more peaceful way of living life. I wish I could be as happy on a daily basis as my son. For that, he is and always will be my inspiration and I will always be his advocate.

There is a wonderful new paradigm of thought I read recently in an evidenced-based research paper by Cheryl Jorgensen, Ph.D. from *Disability Solutions*. (Jorgensen, 2005). She referenced Anne Donnellan, a special education researcher, who wrote that "the criterion of least dangerous assumption holds that in the absence of conclusive data, educational decisions ought to be based on assumptions which, if incorrect, will have the least dangerous effect on the likelihood that students will be able to function independently as adults." Furthermore, she concluded "we should assume that poor performance is due to instructional inadequacy rather than to student deficits" (Donnellan 1984).

Therefore, as Dr. Jorgensen summarized "for Donnellan, the least-dangerous assumption when working with children with severe disabilities is to assume that they are competent and able to learn, because to do otherwise would result in harm such as fewer educational opportunities, inferior literacy instruction, a segregated education, and fewer choices as an adult" (Jorgensen 2005).

After reading this research paper, the thoughts began to create a wonderful new paradigm in my mind where this applied to every single student, not just those with disabilities. We would assume every child could learn and be taught, and every teacher would assume that there was something they could have done differently in their teaching rather than basing it on the deficiency of the child.

Perhaps there were different teaching methods I could have been using to help Taylor with his potty training, feeding issues, and sensory aversions. Maybe it was me. Instead of looking at all of the things Taylor couldn't do, I began to focus on the things he could do if I just changed my approach in teaching him. It was all beginning to make sense, and becoming easier to digest because I had the ability to teach him. The best part of all was that without the negativity of the past draining all of my energy, I could finally concentrate on the important things in my son's life. There truly was a greater calling for Taylor and me. To learn, teach, advocate, and most of all enjoy the journey that made us who we both are today; I've never been prouder: of myself as a mother, and, more importantly, an extraordinary child named Taylor.

References

Donnellan, A. (1984). The criterion of the least dangerous assumption. *Behavioral Disorders, 9*, 141-150.

Jorgensen C. (2005). The least dangerous assumption: A challenge to create a new paradigm. *Disability Solutions, 6*(3), 1, 5-9, 15.